First Aid and Emergency Medicine

First Aid and Emergency Medicine

Edited by
Oscar Cross

Larsen & Keller
www.larsen-keller.com

First Aid and Emergency Medicine
Edited by Oscar Cross
ISBN: 978-1-63549-708-3 (Hardback)

© 2018 Larsen & Keller

▤ Larsen & Keller

Published by Larsen and Keller Education,
5 Penn Plaza,
19th Floor,
New York, NY 10001, USA

Cataloging-in-Publication Data

First aid and emergency medicine / edited by Oscar Cross.
    p. cm.
Includes bibliographical references and index.
ISBN 978-1-63549-708-3
1. First aid in illness and injury. 2. Emergency medicine. I. Cross, Oscar.
RC86.7 .F57 2018
616.025--dc23

For more information regarding Larsen and Keller Education and its products, please visit the publisher's website www.larsen-keller.com

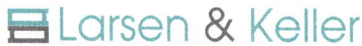

Table of Contents

Permissions

Index

Preface

Emergency medicine refers to the practice of providing immediate treatment and care to people who need instant medical attention. Emergency first aid is the instant first aid provided to people in situations that demand urgent care and treatment. Emergencies usually occur in road accidents, in the cases of sudden heart attack or seizures, organ failures, etc. This book provides comprehensive insights into the field of first aid and emergency medicine. It talks in detail about the various concepts and practices used in this field. Those in search of information to further their knowledge will be greatly assisted by this textbook.

Given below is the chapter wise description of the book:

Chapter 1- The medical aid given to a person injured or suffering from a sudden illness is known as first aid. The training related to first aid can be given in school or public gatherings. The main goal of first aid is to preserve life, prevent further harm and promote recovery. This chapter will provide an integrated understanding of first aid.

Chapter 2- Combat medics are the armed forces who are trained and tasked in providing first aid in times of war. Combat support hospitals can be transported to the war site via aircrafts and then can be reassembled by the staff. First aid and emergency medicine is best understood in confluence with the major topics listed in the following chapter.

Chapter 3- Medical emergencies are sudden or acute illnesses that can result in long-term injury and even death of a person. Depending on the extent of the injury, it may require different levels of medical attention. The emergencies discussed in this section are head injury, coma, bleeding, wound, cardiac tamponade and stroke. The major categories of medical emergencies are dealt with great details in the chapter.

Chapter 4- The immediate medical attention given to patients suffering from illness and injury is known as emergency medicine. There are various models of emergency medicine across the world. The two commonly used models are specialist model and multidisciplinary model. This chapter has been carefully written to provide an easy understanding of the varied aspects of emergency medicine.

Chapter 5- Spinal board is a device used to carry a patient with spinal or limb injuries. It is designed with the purpose of providing rigid support to the patient. The other medical equipment mentioned are automated external defibrillator, autopulse, cervical collar, splint, vacuum mattress, etc. This chapter is an overview of the subject matter incorporating all the major aspects of first aid and emergency medicine.

At the end, I would like to thank all those who dedicated their time and efforts for the successful completion of this book. I also wish to convey my gratitude towards my friends and family who supported me at every step.

Editor

An Introduction to First Aid

The medical aid given to a person injured or suffering from a sudden illness is known as first aid. The training related to first aid can be given in school or public gatherings. The main goal of first aid is to preserve life, prevent further harm and promote recovery. This chapter will provide an integrated understanding of first aid.

First Aid

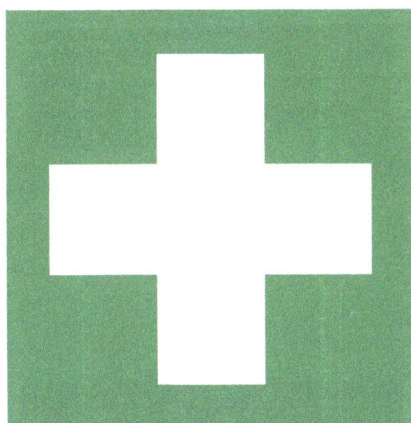

The universal first aid symbol

First aid is the assistance given to any person suffering a sudden illness or injury, with care provided to preserve life, prevent the condition from worsening, and/or promote recovery. It includes initial intervention in a serious condition prior to professional medical help being available, such as performing CPR while awaiting an ambulance, as well as the complete treatment of minor conditions, such as applying a plaster to a cut. First aid is generally performed by the layperson, with many people trained in providing basic levels of first aid, and others willing to do so from acquired knowledge. Mental health first aid is an extension of the concept of first aid to cover mental health.

There are many situations which may require first aid, and many countries have legislation, regulation, or guidance which specifies a minimum level of first aid provision in certain circumstances. This can include specific training or equipment to be available in the workplace (such as an Automated External Defibrillator), the provision of specialist first aid cover at public gatherings, or mandatory first aid training within schools. First aid, however, does not necessarily require any particular equipment or prior knowledge, and can involve improvisation with materials available at the time, often by untrained persons.

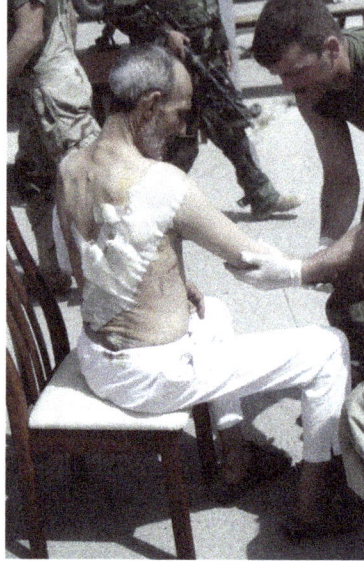

A US Navy corpsman gives first aid to an injured Iraqi citizen.

First aid can be performed on all mammals, although here it relates to the care of human patients.

History

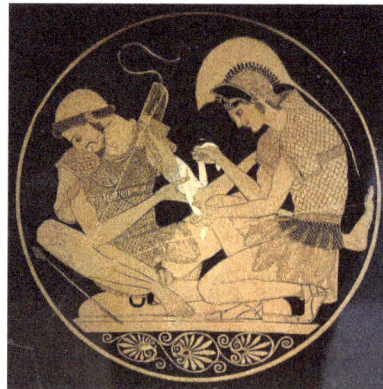

The binding of a battlefield wound depicted on ancient Greek pottery

Early History and Warfare

Skills of what is now known as first aid have been recorded throughout history, especially in relation to warfare, where the care of both traumatic and medical cases is required in particularly large numbers. The Ancient Egyptians (aka people of KMT) were the first to use bandages including the high genius doctor Imhotep. They not only used them to create mummies but also as part of the treatments for surgical patients. Most ancient Greek doctors, philosophers, etc studied in ancient Egypt and then returned to Greece. The bandaging of battle wounds is shown on Classical Greek pottery from circa 500 BCE, whilst the parable of the Good Samaritan includes references to binding or dressing wounds. There are numerous references to first aid performed within the Roman army, with a system of first aid supported by surgeons, field ambulances, and hospitals. Roman legions had the specific role of capsarii, who were responsible for first aid such as bandaging, and are the forerunners of the modern combat medic.

Further examples occur through history, still mostly related to battle, with examples such as the Knights Hospitaller in the 11th century CE, providing care to pilgrims and knights in the Holy Land.

Formalization of Life Saving Treatments

During the late 18th century, drowning as a cause of death was a major concern amongst the population. In 1767, a society for the preservation of life from accidents in water was started in Amsterdam, and in 1773, physician William Hawes began publicizing the power of artificial respiration as means of resuscitation of those who appeared drowned. This led to the formation, in 1774, of the Society for the Recovery of Persons Apparently Drowned, later the Royal Humane Society, who did much to promote resuscitation.

Napoleon's surgeon, Baron Dominique-Jean Larrey, is credited with creating an ambulance corps (the ambulance volantes), which included medical assistants, tasked to administer first aid in battle.

In 1859 Jean-Henri Dunant witnessed the aftermath of the Battle of Solferino, and his work led to the formation of the Red Cross, with a key stated aim of "aid to sick and wounded soldiers in the field". The Red Cross and Red Crescent are still the largest provider of first aid worldwide.

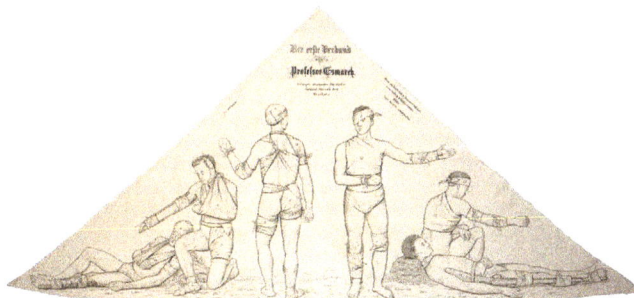

Esmarch bandage showing soldiers how to perform first aid

In 1870, Prussian military surgeon Friedrich von Esmarch introduced formalized first aid to the military, and first coined the term "erste hilfe" (translating to 'first aid'), including training for soldiers in the Franco-Prussian War on care for wounded comrades using pre-learnt bandaging and splinting skills, and making use of the Esmarch bandage which he designed. The bandage was issued as standard to the Prussian combatants, and also included aide-memoire pictures showing common uses.

In 1872, the Order of Saint John of Jerusalem in England changed its focus from hospice care, and set out to start a system of practical medical help, starting with making a grant towards the establishment of the UK's first ambulance service. This was followed by creating its own wheeled transport litter in 1875 (the St John Ambulance), and in 1877 established the St John Ambulance Association (the forerunner of modern-day St John Ambulance) "to train men and women for the benefit of the sick and wounded".

Also in the UK, Surgeon-Major Peter Shepherd had seen the advantages of von Esmarch's new teaching of first aid, and introduced an equivalent programme for the British Army, and so being the first user of "first aid for the injured" in English, disseminating information through a series of lectures. Following this, in 1878, Shepherd and Colonel Francis Duncan took advantage of the newly charitable focus of St John, and established the concept of teaching first aid skills to civilians. The first classes were conducted in the hall of the Presbyterian school in Woolwich (near Woolwich barracks where Shepherd was based) using a comprehensive first aid curriculum.

First aid training began to spread through the British Empire through organisations such as St John, often starting, as in the UK, with high risk activities such as ports and railways.

Aims

The key aims of first aid can be summarised in three key points, sometimes known as 'the three P's':-

- Preserve life: The overriding aim of all medical care which includes first aid, is to save lives and minimize the threat of death.

- Prevent further harm: Prevent further harm also sometimes called prevent the condition from worsening, or danger of further injury, this covers both external factors, such as moving a patient away from any cause of harm, and applying first aid techniques to prevent worsening of the condition, such as applying pressure to stop a bleed becoming dangerous.

- Promote recovery: First aid also involves trying to start the recovery process from the illness or injury, and in some cases might involve completing a treatment, such as in the case of applying a plaster to a small wound.

Key Skills

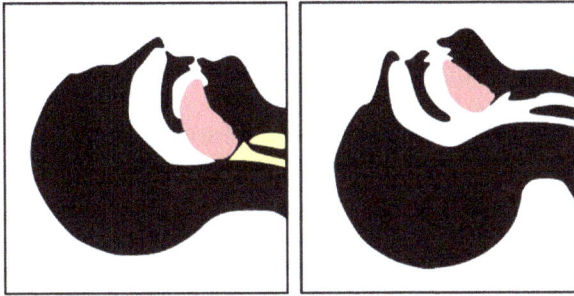

In case of tongue fallen backwards, blocking the airway, it is necessary to hyperextend the head and pull up the chin, so that the tongue lifts and clears the airway.

Certain skills are considered essential to the provision of first aid and are taught ubiquitously. Particularly the "ABC"s of first aid, which focus on critical life-saving intervention, must be rendered before treatment of less serious injuries. ABC stands for *Airway, Breathing,* and *Circulation.* The same mnemonic is used by all emergency health professionals. Attention must first be brought to the airway to ensure it is clear. Obstruction (choking) is a life-threatening emergency. Following evaluation of the airway, a first aid attendant would determine adequacy of breathing and provide rescue breathing if necessary. Assessment of circulation is now not usually carried out for patients who are not breathing, with first aiders now trained to go straight to chest compressions (and thus providing artificial circulation) but pulse checks may be done on less serious patients.

Some organizations add a fourth step of "D" for *Deadly bleeding* or *Defibrillation,* while others consider this as part of the *Circulation* step. Variations on techniques to evaluate and maintain the ABCs depend on the skill level of the first aider. Once the ABCs are secured, first aiders can begin additional treatments, as required. Some organizations teach the same order of priority using the "3Bs": *Breathing, Bleeding,* and *Bones* (or "4Bs": *Breathing, Bleeding, Burns,* and *Bones*). While the ABCs and 3Bs are taught to be performed sequentially, certain conditions may require the consideration of two steps simultaneously. This includes the provision of both artificial respiration and chest compressions to someone who is not breathing and has no pulse, and the consideration of cervical spine injuries when ensuring an open airway.

Preserving Life

In order to stay alive, all persons need to have an open airway—a clear passage where air can move in through the mouth or nose through the pharynx and down into the lungs, without obstruction. Conscious people will maintain their own airway automatically, but those who are unconscious (with a GCS of less than 8) may be unable to maintain a patent airway, as the part of the brain which automatically controls breathing in normal situations may not be functioning.

If the patient was breathing, a first aider would normally then place them in the recovery position, with the patient leant over on their side, which also has the effect of clearing the tongue from the pharynx. It also avoids a common cause of death in unconscious patients, which is choking on regurgitated stomach contents.

The airway can also become blocked through a foreign object becoming lodged in the pharynx or larynx, commonly called choking. The first aider will be taught to deal with this through a combination of 'back slaps' and 'abdominal thrusts'.

Once the airway has been opened, the first aider would assess to see if the patient is breathing. If there is no breathing, or the patient is not breathing normally, such as agonal breathing, the first aider would undertake what is probably the most recognized first aid procedure—cardiopulmonary resuscitation or CPR, which involves breathing for the patient, and manually massaging the heart to promote blood flow around the body.

Promoting Recovery

The first aider is also likely to be trained in dealing with injuries such as cuts, grazes or bone fracture. They may be able to deal with the situation in its entirety (a small adhesive bandage on a paper cut), or may be required to maintain the condition of something like a broken bone, until the next stage of definitive care (usually an ambulance) arrives.

Training

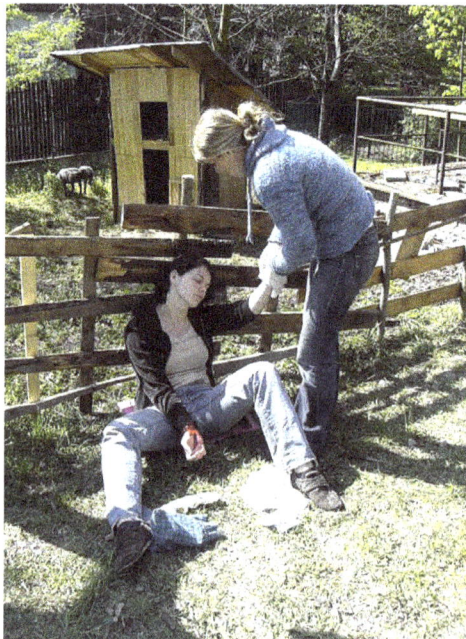

First aid scenario training in progress

Basic principles, such as knowing to use an adhesive bandage or applying direct pressure on a bleed, are often acquired passively through life experiences. However, to provide effective, life-saving first aid interventions requires instruction and practical training. This is especially true where it relates to potentially fatal illnesses and injuries, such as those that require cardiopulmonary resuscitation (CPR); these procedures may be invasive, and carry a risk of further injury to the patient and the provider. As with any training, it is more useful if it occurs *before* an actual emergency, and in many countries, emergency ambulance dispatchers may give basic first aid instructions over the phone while the ambulance is on the way.

Training is generally provided by attending a course, typically leading to certification. Due to regular changes in procedures and protocols, based on updated clinical knowledge, and to maintain skill, attendance at regular refresher courses or re-certification is often necessary. First aid training is often available through community organizations such as the Red Cross and St. John Ambulance, or through commercial providers, who will train people for a fee. This commercial training is most common for training of employees to perform first aid in their workplace. Many community organizations also provide a commercial service, which complements their community programmes.

Specific Disciplines

There are several types of first aid (and first aider) which require specific additional training. These are usually undertaken to fulfill the demands of the work or activity undertaken.

- Aquatic/Marine first aid is usually practiced by professionals such as lifeguards, professional mariners or in diver rescue, and covers the specific problems which may be faced after water-based rescue and/or delayed MedEvac.

- Battlefield first aid takes into account the specific needs of treating wounded combatants and non-combatants during armed conflict.

- Hyperbaric first aid may be practiced by SCUBA diving professionals, who need to treat conditions such as the bends.

- Oxygen first aid is the providing of oxygen to casualties who suffer from conditions resulting in hypoxia.

- Wilderness first aid is the provision of first aid under conditions where the arrival of emergency responders or the evacuation of an injured person may be delayed due to constraints of terrain, weather, and available persons or equipment. It may be necessary to care for an injured person for several hours or days.

- Mental health first aid is taught independently of physical first aid. How to support someone experiencing a mental health problem or in a crisis situation. Also how to identify the first signs of someone developing mental ill health and guide people towards appropriate help.

First Aid Services

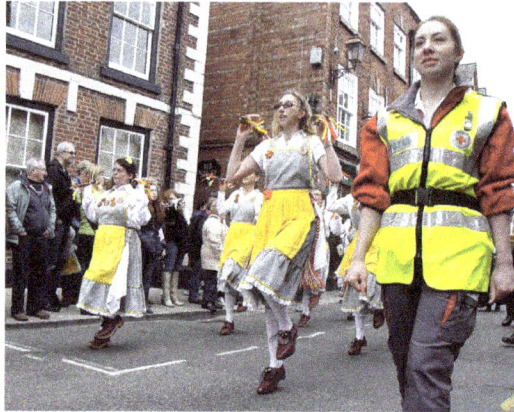

First aider of the British Red Cross accompanies parade of morris dancers
at the Knutsford Royal May Day 2012

Some people undertake specific training in order to provide first aid at public or private events, during filming, or other places where people gather. They may be designated as a first aider, or use some other title. This role may be undertaken on a voluntary basis, with organisations such as the Red Cross and St John Ambulance, or as paid employment with a medical contractor.

People performing a first aid role, whether in a professional or voluntary capacity, are often expected to have a high level of first aid training and are often uniformed.

Symbols

Although commonly associated with first aid, the symbol of a red cross is an official protective symbol of the Red Cross. According to the Geneva Conventions and other international laws, the use of this and similar symbols is reserved for official agencies of the International Red Cross and Red Crescent, and as a protective emblem for medical personnel and facilities in combat situations. Use by any other person or organization is illegal, and may lead to prosecution.

The internationally accepted symbol for first aid is the white cross on a green background.

Some organizations may make use of the Star of Life, although this is usually reserved for use by ambulance services, or may use symbols such as the Maltese Cross, like the Order of Malta Ambulance Corps and St John Ambulance. Other symbols may also be used.

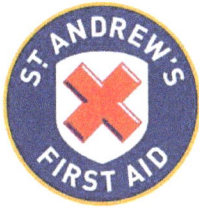
St. Andrew's First Aid Badge

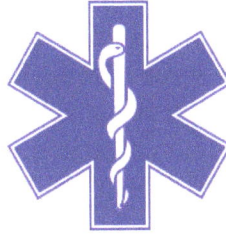
Star of life

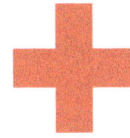
Emblem of the Red Cross

Conditions that Often Require First Aid

- Altitude sickness, which can begin in susceptible people at altitudes as low as 5,000 feet, can cause potentially fatal swelling of the brain or lungs.

- Anaphylaxis, a life-threatening condition in which the airway can become constricted and the patient may go into shock. The reaction can be caused by a systemic allergic reaction to allergens such as insect bites or peanuts. Anaphylaxis is initially treated with injection of epinephrine.

- Battlefield first aid—This protocol refers to treating shrapnel, gunshot wounds, burns, bone fractures, etc. as seen either in the 'traditional' battlefield setting or in an area subject to damage by large-scale weaponry, such as a bomb blast.

- Bone fracture, a break in a bone initially treated by stabilizing the fracture with a splint.

- Burns, which can result in damage to tissues and loss of body fluids through the burn site.

- Cardiac Arrest, which will lead to death unless CPR preferably combined with an AED is started within minutes. There is often no time to wait for the emergency services to arrive as 92 percent of people suffering a sudden cardiac arrest die before reaching hospital according to the American Heart Association.

- Choking, blockage of the airway which can quickly result in death due to lack of oxygen if the patient's trachea is not cleared, for example by the Heimlich Maneuver.

- Childbirth.

- Cramps in muscles due to lactic acid build up caused either by inadequate oxygenation of muscle or lack of water or salt.

- Diving disorders, drowning or asphyxiation.

- Gender-specific conditions, such as dysmenorrhea and testicular torsion.

- Heart attack, or inadequate blood flow to the blood vessels supplying the heart muscle.

- Heat stroke, also known as sunstroke or hyperthermia, which tends to occur during heavy exercise in high humidity, or with inadequate water, though it may occur spontaneously in some chronically ill persons. Sunstroke, especially when the victim has been unconscious, often causes major damage to body systems such as brain, kidney, liver, gastric tract. Unconsciousness for more than two hours usually leads to permanent disability. Emergency treatment involves rapid cooling of the patient.

- Hair tourniquet a condition where a hair or other thread becomes tied around a toe or finger tightly enough to cut off blood flow.

- Heat syncope, another stage in the same process as heat stroke, occurs under similar conditions as heat stroke and is not distinguished from the latter by some authorities.

- Heavy bleeding, treated by applying pressure (manually and later with a pressure bandage) to the wound site and elevating the limb if possible.

- Hyperglycemia (diabetic coma) and Hypoglycemia (insulin shock).

- Hypothermia, or Exposure, occurs when a person's core body temperature falls below 33.7 °C (92.6 °F). First aid for a mildly hypothermic patient includes rewarming, which can be achieved by wrapping the affected person in a blanket, and providing warm drinks, such as soup, and high energy food, such as chocolate. However, rewarming a severely hypothermic person could result in a fatal arrhythmia, an irregular heart rhythm.

- Insect and animal bites and stings.

- Joint dislocation.

- Poisoning, which can occur by injection, inhalation, absorption, or ingestion.

- Seizures, or a malfunction in the electrical activity in the brain. Three types of seizures include a grand mal (which usually features convulsions as well as temporary respiratory abnormalities, change in skin complexion, etc.) and petit mal (which usually features twitching, rapid blinking, and/or fidgeting as well as altered consciousness and temporary respiratory abnormalities).

- Muscle strains and Sprains, a temporary dislocation of a joint that immediately reduces automatically but may result in ligament damage.

- Stroke, a temporary loss of blood supply to the brain.

- Toothache, which can result in severe pain and loss of the tooth but is rarely life-threatening, unless over time the infection spreads into the bone of the jaw and starts osteomyelitis.

- Wounds and bleeding, including lacerations, incisions and abrasions, Gastro-intestinal bleeding, avulsions and Sucking chest wounds, treated with an occlusive dressing to let air out but not in.

First Aid Kit

Many accidents can happen at home, office, schools, laboratories etc. which require immediate attention before the patient is attended by the doctor.

Making of the First Aid Kit

Though professional first aid kits are readily available one can make a simple kit easily at home. Still ready made First Aid kits/boxes/pouches/cases are recommended as they have well organized compartments. To make a First Aid kit, a strong, durable bag or transparent plastic box should be taken and a white cross in a green square placed on the sides and on the top. This will make for easy identification of the box to any user. The kit should be kept such that it is within reach in case of an emergency.

A First Aid Kit should have the following contents:

- first-aid manual different sizes
- adhesive tape
- adhesive bandages in severe sizes
- elastic bandage
- a splint
- antiseptic wipes
- soap
- antibiotic ointment
- antiseptic solution (like hydrogen peroxide or saline)
- hydrocortisone cream (1%)
- acetaminophen and ibuprofen
- extra prescription medications (if the family is going on vacation)
- tweezers
- sharp scissors

- safety pins

- disposable instant cold packs

- calamine lotion

- alcohol wipes or ethyl alcohol

- thermometer

- tooth preservation kit

- plastic non-latex gloves(at least 2 pairs)

- flashlight and extra batteries

- thermal shock blanket

- mouthpiece for administering CPR (can be obtained from your local Red Cross)

- blanket (stored nearby)

- First Aid Card containing emergency personal information, phone numbers, medications, manual.

Aid Station

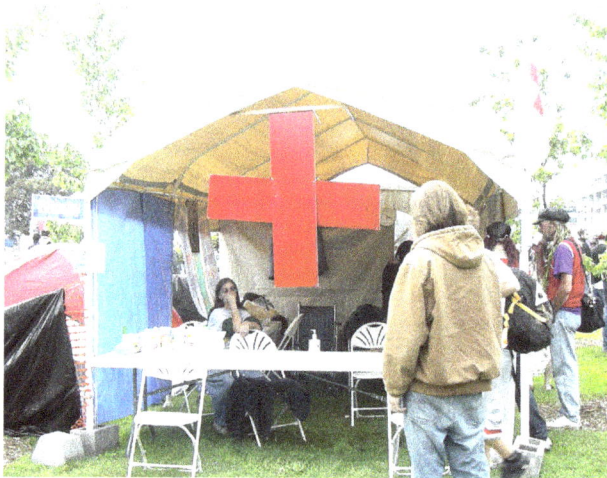

An aid station at a public festival.

An aid station is a temporary facility (often a tent, table, or general rest area) established to provide supplies to endurance event participants or medical first aid and provisions during major events, disaster response situations, or military operations.

Aid stations may be divided into sections where the station serves both medical and non-medical functions.

Sporting Events

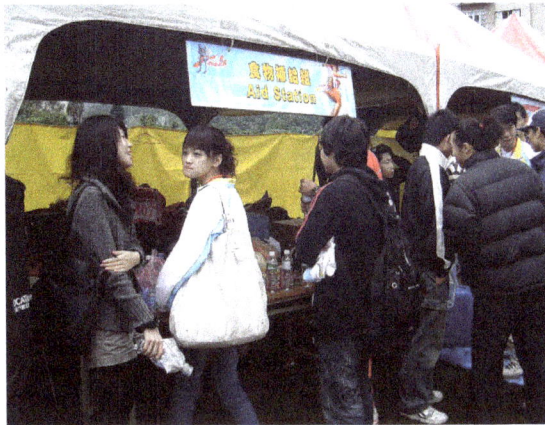

An aid station at the 2007 Soochow 24-hour ultramarathon.

At endurance races like marathons or bicycle racing events, aid stations are established along the race route to provide supplies (food, water, and repair equipment) to participants. During modern cycle races, aid station functions may be performed by a mobile SAG Wagon (*"Supplies And Gear"*) or support vehicle that travels with participants at the rear of the *peloton*.

Typically sports drinks and energy gels are provided as well as water. Depending on the length of the race, food may be available. Often, medical supplies will also be available.

The aid station may also serve as a checkpoint to track competitors. During events where the distance between aid stations is predetermined and known by competitors, some trainers advise using aid stations as course markers for pace-setting.

At some major annual marathon events, particular aid stations and their operators have become local institutions. The Chicago Marathon, for example, has annual prizes for aid stations and aid station volunteers and some volunteers have managed the same station each year for many years. The event includes very large stations, some with more than 300 volunteers, and event organisers publish an *Aid Station Instruction Book*.

Military Operations

During combat or training operations, military units may establish aid stations behind front lines to provide medical support to troops in the field. In United States military operations, these are most commonly referred to as Battalion Aid Stations; in Commonwealth countries, Regimental Aid Posts. The term "Main Aid Station" is also used depending on size and operational context. Aid stations are the smallest units, passing cases on to Field Ambulances and thence to Casualty clearing stations.

During the Napoleonic Wars (1803–1815), the French established a tiered system of medical support services. Basic aid stations operated by one field medic were established as close to front lines as possible, sometimes within a few hundred meters to allow for the treatment of wounded troops as soon as possible. The more seriously injured were transported further back behind front lines to field hospitals in churches or nearby chateaus. Those who required more extensive treatment were transported again to much larger permanent "receiving" military hospitals in France.

Aid stations may also be established during training operations where the deployment of a "full hospital" is not required and the injuries treated are not as severe as those experienced during combat operations. In such situations, aid station medics provide "level one" care and treatment of non-life-threatening injuries or illness. There is generally no provision for treating "serious or life-threatening" problems beyond stabilization for transportation to a larger medical facility.

Disaster Response

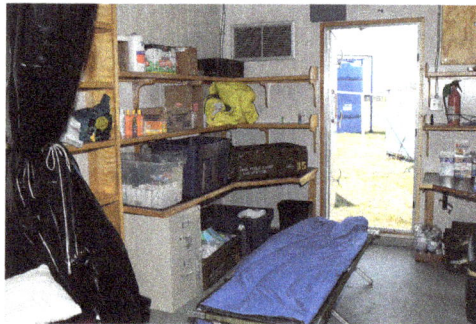

A temporary Federal Emergency Management Agency aid station.

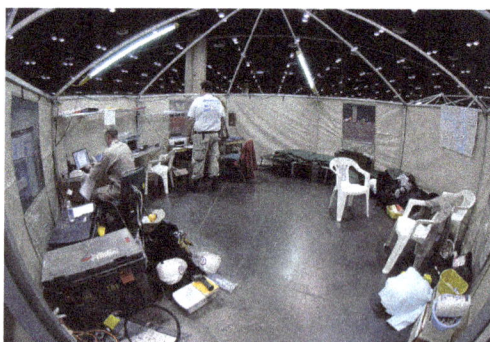

Inside a Disaster Medical Assistance Team aid station.

In disaster areas, aid stations may be established to provide triage for injured persons or longer term support for those in need of food or shelter.

Aid stations may be established in response to both a natural and man-made disaster events and may remain in place for the duration of the disaster recovery effort or may be replaced by larger or more permanent facilities. William L. Waugh gives the example of an aid station established during the aftermath of the Hyatt Regency walkway collapse and later replaced with more substantive triage facilities.

In the immediate aftermath of Hurricane Katrina, FEMA and the Red Cross established a number of emergency aid stations throughout New Orleans and near evacuation centers. These provided food, water, recovery supplies, medical aid and became a focal point of efforts to find missing persons. A number of privately owned facilities became makeshift aid stations including the bar, *Johnny White's*.

Understanding Combat Medic

Combat medics are the armed forces who are trained and tasked in providing first aid in times of war. Combat support hospitals can be transported to the war site via aircrafts and then can be reassembled by the staff. First aid and emergency medicine is best understood in confluence with the major topics listed in the following chapter.

Military Medicine

The term military medicine has a number of potential connotations. It may mean:

- A medical specialty, specifically a branch of occupational medicine attending to the medical risks and needs (both preventive and interventional) of soldiers, sailors and other service members. This disparate arena has historically involved the prevention and treatment of infectious diseases (especially tropical diseases), and, in the 20th Century, the ergonomics and health effects of operating military-specific machines and equipment such as submarines, tanks, helicopters and airplanes. Undersea and aviation medicine can be understood as subspecialties of military medicine, or in any case originated as such. Few countries certify or recognize "military medicine" as a formal speciality or subspeciality in its own right.

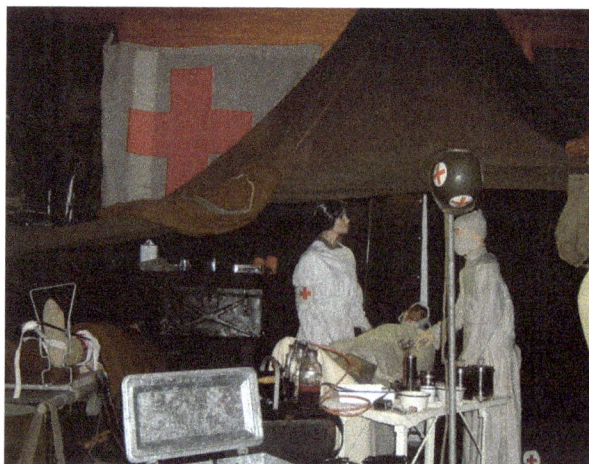

WWII era field hospital re-created operating tent using puppets, Diekirch Military Museum, Luxembourg

- The planning and practice of the surgical management of mass battlefield casualties and the logistical and administrative considerations of establishing and operating combat support hospitals. This involves military medical hierarchies, especially the organization of structured medical command and administrative systems that interact with and support deployed combat units.

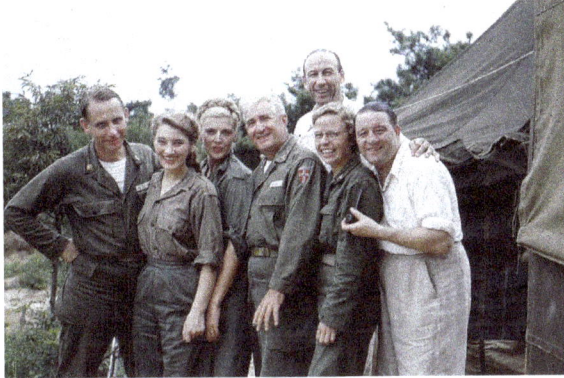
Norwegian NORMASH personnel during the Korean War

- The administration and practice of health care for military service members and their dependents in non-deployed (peacetime) settings. This may (as in the United States) consist of a medical system paralleling all the medical specialties and sub-specialties that exist in the civilian sector.

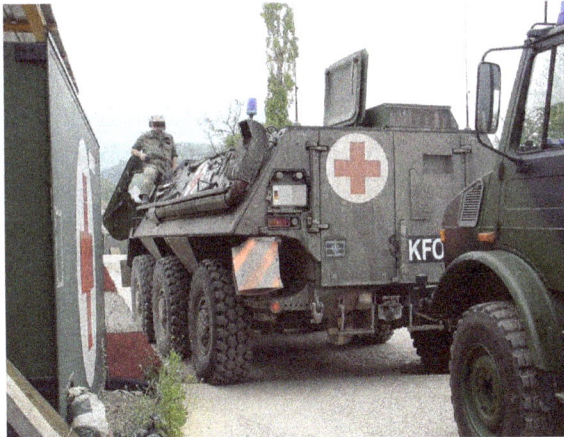
German Kosovo Force armoured medical transport, marked with the protective sign

- Medical research and development specifically bearing upon problems of military medical interest. Historically, this encompasses all of the medical advances emerging from medical research efforts directed at addressing the problems encountered by deployed military forces (e.g., vaccines or drugs for soldiers, medical evacuation systems, drinking water chlorination, etc.) many of which ultimately prove important beyond the purely military considerations that inspired them.

Legal Status

Military medical personnel engage in humanitarian work and are "protected persons" under international humanitarian law in accordance with the First and Second Geneva Conventions and their Additional Protocols, which established legally binding rules guaranteeing neutrality and protection for wounded soldiers, field or ship's medical personnel, and specific humanitarian institutions in an armed conflict. International humanitarian law makes no distinction between medical personnel who are members of the armed forces (and who hold military ranks) and those who are civilian volunteers. All medical personnel are considered non-combatants under international humanitarian law because of their humanitarian duties, and they may not be attacked and not be taken as prisoners of war; hospitals and other medical facilities and transports identified as such, whether they are military or civilian, may not be attacked either. The red cross, the red crescent and the red crystal are the protective signs recognised under international humanitarian law, and are used by military medical personnel and facilities for this purpose. Attacking military medical personnel, patients in their care, or medical facilities or transports legitimately marked as such is a war crime. Likewise, misusing these protective signs to mask military operations is the war crime of perfidy. Military medical personnel may be armed, usually with service pistols, for the purpose of self defense or the defense of patients.

Historical Significance

The significance of military medicine for combat strength goes far beyond treatment of battlefield injuries; in every major war fought until the late 19th century disease claimed more soldier casualties than did enemy action. During the American Civil War (1860–65), for example, about twice as many soldiers died of disease as were killed or mortally wounded in combat. The Franco-Prussian War (1870–71) is considered to have been the first conflict in which combat injury exceeded disease, at least in the German coalition army which lost 3.47% of its average headcount to combat and only 1.82% to disease. In new world countries, such as Australia, New Zealand, the United States and Canada, military physicians and surgeons contributed significantly to the development of civilian health care.

Improvements in military medicine have increased the survival rates in successive wars, due to improvements in medical evacuation, battlefield medicine and trauma care. Similar improvements have been seen in the trauma practices during the Iraq war. Some military trauma care practices are disseminated by citizen soldiers who return to civilian practice. One such practice is where major trauma patients are transferred to an operating theater as soon as possible, to stop internal bleeding, increasing the survival rate. Within the United States, the survival rate for gunshot wounds has increased, leading to apparent declines in the gun death rate in states that have stable rates of gunshot hospitalizations.

North America

Canada

- Royal Canadian Medical Service
- Royal Canadian Dental Corps
- Canadian Forces Health Services Group
- Surgeon General (Canada)

United States

- Military Health System
- *Military Medicine*, academic journal
- TRICARE
- Uniformed Services University of the Health Sciences
- Henry M. Jackson Foundation for the Advancement of Military Medicine
- Defense Health Agency
- Joint Task Force National Capital Region/Medical
- Executive Order 13139
- Professional Medical Film

U.S. Army

- 68W, the "combat medic"
- Army Medical Department
- Battalion Aid Stations
- Borden Institute
- Combat Support Hospital
- Fort Detrick
- Fort Sam Houston
- Forward Surgical Teams
- Medical Corps (United States Army)
- Nurse Corps (United States Army)
- Mobile Army Surgical Hospital

- Surgeon General of the U.S. Army
- *Textbook of Military Medicine* (1989–2007), published by the U.S. Army
- U.S. Army Dental Command
- U.S. Army Medical Command

U.S. Navy

- Surgeon General of the U.S. Navy
- U.S. Navy Dental Corps
- U.S. Navy Hospital Corpsman
- U.S. Navy Medical Corps
- U.S. Navy Medical Service Corps
- U.S. Navy Nurse Corps
- Naval Medical Center San Diego
- Naval Medical Center Portsmouth
- National Naval Medical Center (now the Walter Reed National Military Medical Center)
- Hospital ship
- Diving medicine

U.S. Air Force

- Surgeon General of the U.S. Air Force
- U.S. Air Force Medical Service (including Dental Corps, Medical Corps, Nursing Corps, and other corps)
- Aeromedical evacuation
- Aviation medicine

Europe

France

- French Defence Health Service

Belgium

- Belgian Medical Component

Germany

- Bundeswehr Joint Medical Service
- Generaloberstabsarzt

Italy

- Corpo sanitario dell'Esercito Italiano
- Corpo sanitario militare marittimo
- Corpo sanitario aeronautico
- Servizio sanitario dell'Arma dei carabinieri

Russia

- Main Military Medical Directorate
- Kirov Military Medical Academy (founded in 1798)
- Military academies in Russia#Kuybyshev Military Medical Academy
- *Military Medical Business*, academic journal
- Museum of Military Medicine

Serbia

- Military Medical Academy

United Kingdom

- Medical Assistant (Royal Navy)
- Royal Navy Medical Service
- Queen Alexandra's Royal Naval Nursing Service
- Queen Alexandra's Royal Army Nursing Corps
- Princess Mary's Royal Air Force Nursing Service
- Army Medical Services
- Royal Army Medical Corps
  - Medical Support Officer
  - Combat Medical Technician

- RAF Medical Services
- Surgeon-General (United Kingdom)
- Defence Medical Services

Other Regions

Australia

- Australian Army Medical Units, World War I
- Royal Australian Army Medical Corps
- Royal Australian Army Nursing Corps

Israel

- Logistics, Medical, and the Centers Directorate
- Medical Corps (Israel)

South Africa

- South African Medical Service

Vietnam

- Vietnam Military Medical University (*Học Viện Quân Y*) in Hanoi

India

Armed Forces Medical College

International

- International Committee of Military Medicine
- Committee of Chiefs of Military Medical Services in NATO (COMEDS)

Battlefield Medicine

Battlefield medicine, also called field surgery and later combat casualty care, is the treatment of wounded combatants and non-combatants in or near an area of combat. Civilian medicine has been greatly advanced by procedures that were first developed to treat the wounds inflicted during combat. With the advent of advanced procedures and medical technology, even polytrauma can be survivable in modern wars. Battlefield medicine is a category of military medicine.

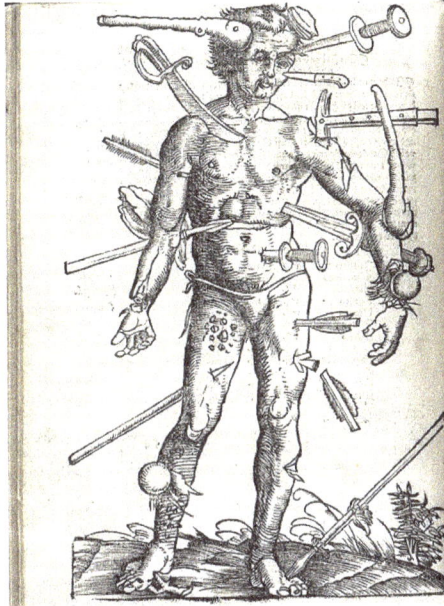

An illustration showing a variety of wounds from the *Feldbuch der Wundarznei* (*Field manual for the treatment of wounds*) by Hans von Gersdorff, (1517); illustration by Hans Wechtlin.

Chronology of Medical Advances on the Battlefield

- During the Battle of Shrewsbury in 1403, Prince Henry had an arrow removed from his face using a specially designed surgical instrument.

- Ambulances or dedicated vehicles for the purpose of carrying injured persons. These were first used by Spanish soldiers during the Siege of Málaga (1487).

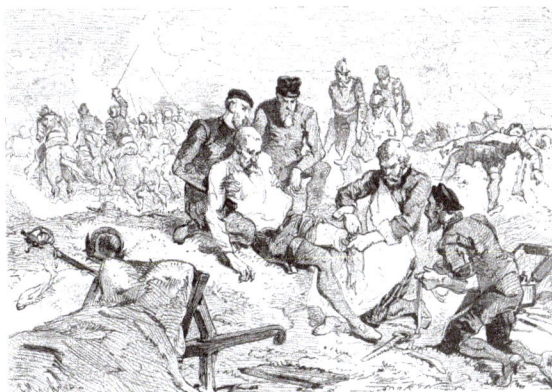

Ambroise Paré, on the battlefield using a ligature for the artery of an amputated leg of a soldier.

- French military surgeon Ambroise Paré (1510–90) pioneered modern battle-field wound treatment. His two main contributions to battlefield medicine are the use of dressing to treat wounds and the use of ligature to stop bleeding during amputation.

- The practice of *triage* pioneered by Dominique Jean Larrey during the Napole-onic Wars (1803–1815). He also pioneered the use of ambulances in the midst of combat ('ambulances volantes', or flying ambulances). Prior to this, military ambulances had waited for combat to cease before collecting the wounded by which time many casualties would have succumbed to their injuries.

- Russian surgeon Nikolay Ivanovich Pirogov was one of the first surgeons to use ether as an anaesthetic in 1847, as well as the very first surgeon to use anaesthe-sia in a field operation during the Crimean War.

- American Civil War surgeon Jonathan Letterman (1824–72) originated mod-ern methods of medical organization within armies.

- Advances in surgery - especially amputation, during the Napoleonic Wars and First World War on the battlefield of the Somme.

- During the Spanish Civil War there were two major advances. The first one was the invention of a practical method for transporting blood. Developed in Bar-celona by Duran i Jordà, the technique mixed the blood of the donors with the same blood type and then, using Grífols glass tubes and a refrigerator truck, transported the blood to the frontline. A few weeks later Norman Bethune de-veloped a similar service. The second advance was the invention of the mobile operating room by the Catalan Moisès Broggi, who worked for the International Brigades.

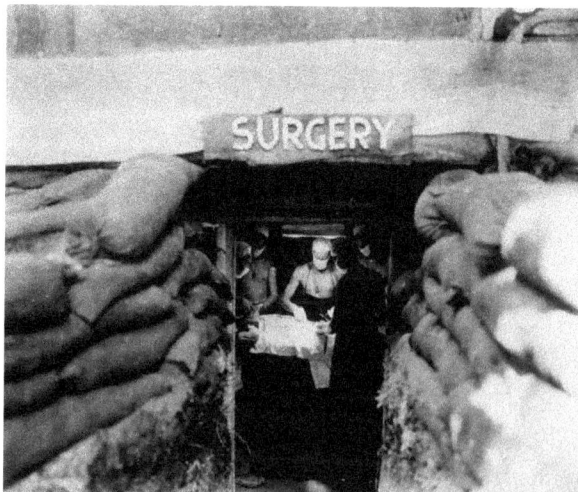

A US Army soldier, wounded by a Japanese sniper, undergoes surgery during the Bougainville Campaign in World War II.

- The establishment of fully equipped and mobile field hospitals such as the Mobile Army Surgical Hospital was first practiced by the United States in World War II. It was succeeded in 2006 by the Combat Support Hospital.

- The use of helicopters as ambulances, or MEDEVACs was first practiced in Burma in 1944. The first medivac under fire was done in Manila in 1945 where over 70 troops were extracted in five helicopters, one and two at a time.

- The extension of emergency medicine to prehospital settings through the use of emergency medical technicians.

- The use of Remote physiological monitoring devices on soldiers to show vital signs and biomechanical data to the medic and MEDEVAC crew before and during trauma. This allows medicine and treatment to be administered as soon as possible in the field and during extraction.

Current Battlefield Medicine used by the U.S Military

Over the past decade combat medicine has improved drastically. Everything has been given a complete overhaul from the training to the gear. In 2011, all enlisted military medical training for the U.S. Navy, Air Force, and Army were located under one command, the Medical Education and Training Campus (METC). After attending a basic medical course there (which is similar to a civilian EMT course), the students go on to advanced training in Tactical Combat Casualty Care.

Tactical Combat Casualty Care

Today, TCCC is becoming the standard of care for the tactical management of combat casualties within the Department of Defense and is the sole standard of care endorsed by both the American College of Surgeons and the National Association of EMT's for casualty management in tactical environments.

TCCC is built around three definitive phases of casualty care:

1. Care Under Fire: Care rendered at the scene of the injury while both the medic and the casualty are under hostile fire. Available medical equipment is limited to that carried by each operator and the medic. This stage focuses on a quick assessment, and placing a tourniquet on any major bleed.

2. Tactical Field Care: Rendered once the casualty is no longer under hostile fire. Medical equipment is still limited to that carried into the field by mission personnel. Time prior to evacuation may range from a few minutes to many hours. Care here may include advanced airway treatment, IV therapy, etc. The treatment rendered varies depending on the skill level of the provider as well as the supplies available. This is when a corpsman/medic will make a triage and evacuation decision.

3. Tactical Evacuation Care (TACEVAC): Rendered while the casualty is evacuated to a higher echelon of care. Any additional personnel and medical equipment pre-staged in these assets will be available during this phase.

Since "90% of combat deaths occur on the battlefield before the casualty ever reaches a medical treatment facility" (Col. Ron Bellamy) TCCC focuses training on major hemorrhaging, and airway complications such as a tension-pneumothorax. This has driven the casualty fatality rate down to less than 9%.

Combat Medic

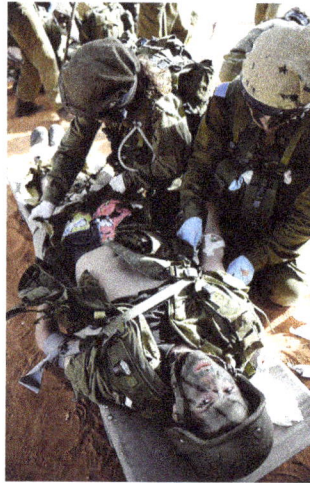

IDF field doctors training in Israel

Combat medics or Field medics (or medics) are military personnel who have been trained to at least an EMT level (16-week course in the U.S. Army), and are responsible for providing first aid and frontline trauma care on the battlefield. They are also responsible for providing continuing medical care in the absence of a readily available physician, including care for disease and battle injuries. Combat medics are normally co-located with the combat troops they serve in order to easily move with the troops and monitor ongoing health.

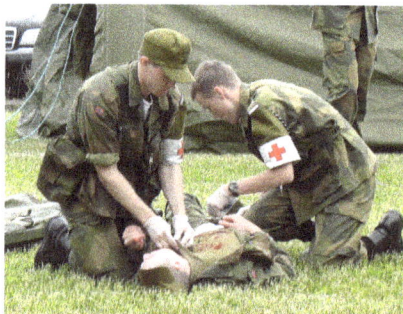

Norwegian medics during an exercise

Geneva Convention Protection

In 1864, sixteen European states adopted the first-ever Geneva Convention to save lives and alleviate the suffering of wounded and sick persons in the battlefield. As well as to protect trained medical personnel as non-combatants, in the act of rendering aid.

Chapter IV, Article 25 of the Geneva Convention states that: "Members of the armed forces specially trained for employment, should the need arise, as hospital orderlies, nurses or auxiliary stretcher-bearers, in the search for or the collection, transport or treatment of the wounded and sick shall likewise be respected and protected if they are carrying out these duties at the time when they come into contact with the enemy or fall into his hands." Article 29 reads: "Members of the personnel designated in Article 25 who have fallen into the hands of the enemy, shall be prisoners of war, but shall be employed on their medical duties insofar as the need arises."

According to the Geneva Convention, knowingly firing at a medic wearing clear insignia is a war crime.

In modern times, most combat medics carry a personal weapon, to be used to protect themselves and the wounded or sick in their care. When and if they use their arms offensively, they then sacrifice their protection under the Geneva Conventions. These medics are specifically trained.

History

Surgeon Dominique Jean Larrey directed the Grande Armée of Napoleon to develop mobile field hospitals, or "ambulances volantes" (flying ambulances), in addition to a corps of trained and equipped soldiers (infirmiers tenues de service) to aid those on the battlefield. Before Larrey's initiative in the 1790s, wounded soldiers were either left amid the fighting until the combat ended or their comrades would carry them to the rear line.

It was during the American Civil War that Surgeon (Major) Jonathan Letterman, Medical Director of the Army of the Potomac, realized a need for an integrated medical treatment and evacuation system. He saw the need to equip this system with its own dedicated vehicles, organizations, facilities, and personnel. The Letterman plan was first implemented in September 1862 at the Battle of Antietam, Maryland.

The United States Army's need for medical and scientific specialty officers to support combat operations resulted in the creation of two temporary components: the U.S. Army Ambulance Service, established on June 23, 1917 and the Sanitary Corps, established on June 30, 1917. Officers of the Sanitary Corps served in medical logistics, hospital administration, patient administration, resource management, x-ray, laboratory engineering, physical reconstruction, gas defense, and venereal disease control. They were dedicated members of the medical team that enabled American generals to concentrate on enemy threats rather than epidemic threats. On August 4, 1947, Congress created the Navy Medical Service Corps.

In the United States, a report entitled "Accidental Death and Disability: The Neglected Disease of Modern Society (1966)", was published by National Academy of Sciences and the National Research Council. Better known as "The White Paper" to emergency providers, it revealed that soldiers who were seriously wounded on the battlefields of Vietnam had a better survival rate than those individuals who were seriously injured in motor vehicle accidents on California freeways. Early research attributed these differences in outcome to a number of factors, including comprehensive trauma care, rapid transport to designated trauma facilities, and a new type of medical corpsman, one who was trained to perform certain critical advanced medical procedures such as fluid replacement and airway management, which allowed the victim to survive the journey to definitive care.

Red Cross, Red Crescent, and MDA

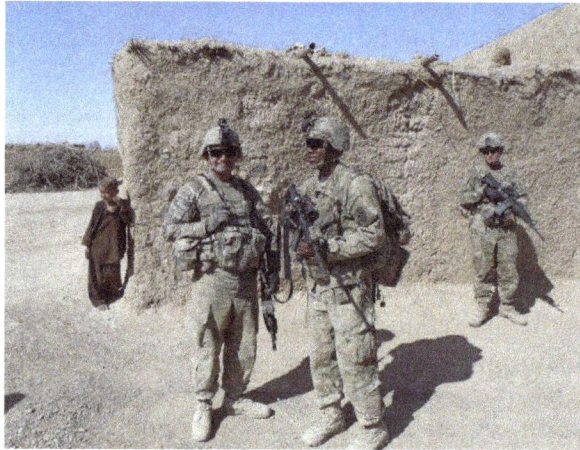

A U.S. Army combat medic (center-right) in Afghanistan. Note that the only distinguishing feature is the medical pack on his back.

The International Committee of the Red Cross, a private humanitarian institution based in Switzerland, provided the first official symbol for medical personnel. The first Geneva convention, originally called for "Amelioration of the Condition of the Wounded and Sick in Armed Forces in the Field," officially adopted the red cross on a field of white as the identifying emblem. This symbol was meant to signify to enemy combatants that the medic qualifies as a non-combatant, at least while providing medical care. Islamic countries use a Red Crescent instead. During the 1876–1878 war between Russia and Turkey, the Ottoman Empire declared that it would use a red crescent instead of a red cross as its emblem, although it agreed to respect the red cross used by the other side. Although these symbols were officially sponsored by the International Federation of Red Cross and Red Crescent Societies, the Magen David Adom ("MDA"), Israel's emergency relief service, used the Magen David (a red star of David on a white background).

Israeli medics still wear the Magen David. To enable MDA to become a fully recognized and participating member of the International Red Cross and Red Crescent Movement, Protocol III was adopted. It is an amendment to the Geneva Conventions relating to the Adoption of an Additional Distinctive Emblem and authorizes the use of a new emblem, known as the third protocol emblem or the Red Crystal. For indicative use on foreign territory, any national society can incorporate its unique symbol into the Red Crystal. Under Protocol III, the MDA will continue to employ the red Magen David for domestic use, and will employ the red crystal on international relief missions.

Modern Day

Medical personnel from most western nations carry weapons for protection of themselves and their patients but remain designated non combatants, wearing the red cross, crescent or crystal.

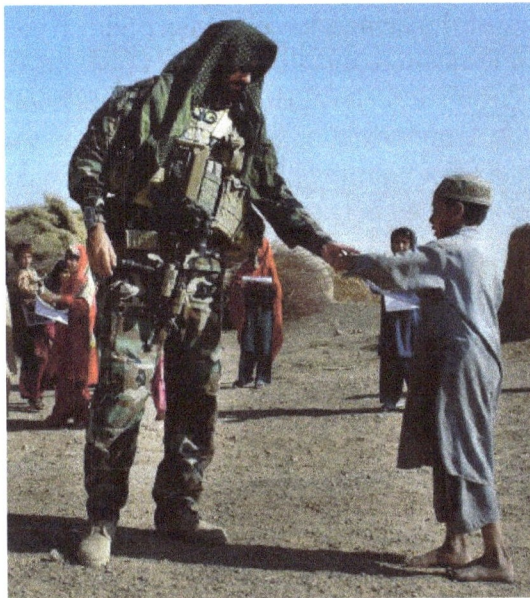

A U.S. Special Forces medic in Afghanistan.

Traditionally, most United States medical personnel also wore a distinguishing red cross, to denote their protection as non-combatants under the Geneva Convention. This practice continued into World War II. However, the enemies faced by professional armies in more recent conflicts are often insurgents who either do not recognize the Geneva Convention, or do not care, and readily engage all personnel, irrespective of non-combatant status. As their non combatant status is not respected, many US medics no longer wear non combatant markings. This can enable medics to be used as medically trained soldiers, fighting aggressively rather than just in self-defence. Combat Medics in the United States Army and United States Navy Hospital Corpsmen are virtually indistinguishable from regular combat troops, except for the extra medical equipment they carry.

In the U.S. Navy, enlisted medical personnel are known as Corpsmen, not medics. The colloquial form of address for a Hospital Corpsman is "Doc." In the U.S. Marine Corps, this term is generally used as a sign of respect. The U.S. Navy deploys FMF Hospital Corpsman attached to U.S. Marine Corps units as part of the Fleet Marine Force. Since the U.S. Marine Corps is part of the Department of the Navy, it relies on Navy Corpsmen and other Naval medical personnel for medical care.

USAF medics have frequently served attached to U.S. Army units in recent conflicts. Though all combat medical personnel are universally referred to as "medic", within different branches of the U.S. military, the skill level, quality of training and scope of work performed by medics varies from branch to branch. The U.S Army commonly addresses Line Medics as "Doc" provided that they have earned the title, as it is not easily earned.

As a result of the 2005 BRAC, the U.S. Department of Defense has moved most medical training for all branches of the armed forces to Fort Sam Houston of Joint Base San Antonio. A new Medical Education and Training Campus was constructed and the Air Force's 937th Training Group and Naval Hospital Corps School were relocated to Fort Sam Houston, joining the Army's existing Army Medical Department Center & School. Although each service has some training particular to its branch, the bulk of the course material and instruction is shared between medical personnel of the different services.

Combat Support Hospital

A combat support hospital (CSH, pronounced "cash") is a type of modern United States military field hospital. The CSH is transportable by aircraft and trucks and is normally delivered to the Corps Support Area in standard military-owned Demountable Containers (MILVAN) cargo containers. Once transported, it is assembled by the staff into a tent hospital to treat patients. Depending upon the operational environment (e.g., battlefield), a CSH might also treat civilians and wounded enemy soldiers. The CSH is the successor to the Mobile Army Surgical Hospital.

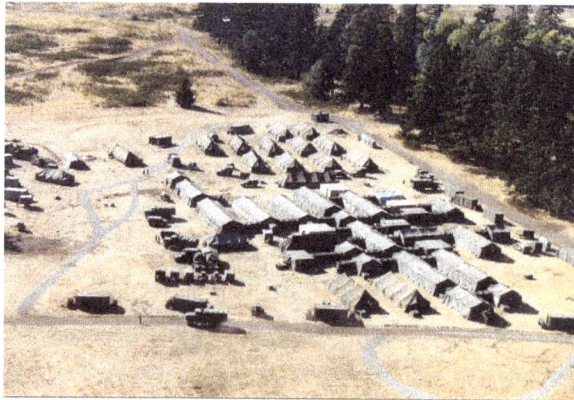

47th Combat Support Hospital at Fort Lewis, Washington, circa 2000.

Facility

The size of a combat support hospital is not limited, since tents can be chained together; it will typically deploy with between 44 and 248 hospital beds, with 44 beds being most common (ATP 4.02-5 Casualty Care, May 2013) For patient care the CSH is climate-controlled, and has pharmacy, laboratory, X-Ray (often including a CT Scanner) and dental capabilities (ATP 4-02.5 Casualty Care, May 2013). It provides its own power from generators.

The great operational advantage of the DEPloyable MEDical Systems (DEPMEDS) facility is the use of single or double expanding ISO containers/units to create hard sided, air conditioned, sterile operating rooms and intensive care facilities, which can produce surgical outcomes similar to that seen in fixed facility hospitals, and do so in an austere environment.

Function

Because they are large and relatively difficult to move, combat support hospitals are not the front line of battlefield medicine. Battalion Aid Stations, Forward Support Medical Battalions and Forward Surgical Teams are usually the first point of contact medical care for wounded soldiers. The CSH receives most patients via helicopter Air Ambulance, and stabilizes these patients for further treatment at fixed facility hospitals. Ideally, the CSH is located as the bridge between incoming helicopter ambulances and outgoing Air Force aircraft.

The CSH is capable of providing definitive care for many cases. Current medical doctrine does not encourage wounded soldiers, if they are not expected to quickly return to operational status, to stay in the combat zone. This is a pragmatic decision as the resources are usually available to bring them home quickly. Military aircraft constantly fly into a theater of operations loaded with equipment and supplies, but often lack a back cargo. Given that adequate "airlift" is usually present, it is easy to evacuate wounded promptly. For this reason the CSH bed capacity is not as heavily used as in past conflicts.

The CSH will generally have a ground ambulance company attached. This company consists of approximately 4 platoons of ground ambulances commanded by a Medical Service Corps officer. The ground ambulance company in cooperation with available air ambulances (MEDEVAC) is responsible for the movement of sick and wounded from the Battalion Aid Station and other forward-deployed locations to the CSH, as well as evacuation through an established medical treatment chain leading ultimately, for those seriously sick or wounded, to hospitals in the Continental United States in cooperation with resources in the U.S. Air Force.

The CSH is larger than its predecessor, the Mobile Army Surgical Hospital. It is commanded by a colonel, rather than a lieutenant colonel.

A fully manned CSH has over 600 people when fully staffed 248 beds. The modular nature of the organization allows for partial deployments, and the full unit is not often deployed (ATP 4.02-5 Casualty Care, May 2013).

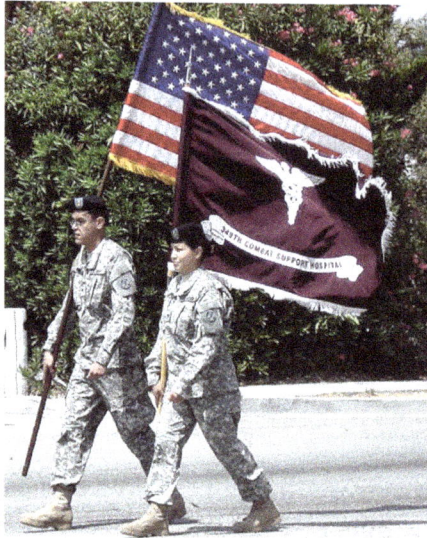

349th CSH unit, marching in the Torrance Armed Forces Day Parade.

History and Past Configurations

In 1973 and 1974, the 28th Surgical Hospital MASH helped phase-in new designs for operating rooms and patient facilities from the previous canvas tents. Since then all other configurations of army deployable hospitals have been inactivated or reconfigured to the CSH configuration. The last to convert was the 212th Mobile Army Surgical Hospital.

In the mid 1970s the "MUST" designation was applied, (Medical Unit, Self Contained, Transportable). During the "Cold War", with the possible conflict with the Warsaw Pact, active duty MUST units would be staffed by all the basic personnel necessary (Medics, X-Ray Techs, Pharmacist, Cooks, Clerks etc.) Doctors, Nurses and Specialist would be mobilized and mate up with the unit in the Field. The Unit would be flown to West Germany, withdraw Pre-positioned complete Hospital MUST equipment and Military Vehicles from warehouses and then deploy. It contained all necessary functions to provide care for 200 beds, including 2 intensive care units, 8 medical wards, emergency room, 4 operating rooms, orthopedic room, laboratory, X-ray, pharmacy and the Unit's transport vehicles. It consisted of hard containers, which would be transported to the designated site, then the wheels would be removed and then expanded. They housed the operating rooms, laboratory, X-ray, and pharmacy. Inflatable shelters were used to provide double wall insulated areas for the patient care areas of the hospital. These "inflatables" required a power system called a Utility Pack (also known as a U-Pack or power station) to provide utility services, Heat, Cooling, Inflation, Hot Water, Filtered Air from CBR Contaminants. The Utility Pack (Power Plant, Utility, Gas Turbine Engine Driven - Libby Welding Co. Model LPU-71, Airesearch Model PPU85-5, AmerTech Co. Model APP-1, or Hollingsworth Model JHTWX10/96), powered by a centrifugal flow gas turbine engine, provided electricity (60 Hz AC, 400 Hz AC, and 24vdc). At 250 beds the hospital required 8 U-Packs. Each consumed 30 gallons of jet fuel per hour. After several years of using inflatables they were abandoned in the mid 1980s, largely due to the weight of the inflatables, and the amount of fuel required just to keep the tents from collapsing.

Combat Medical Technician

A combat medical technician (CMT) is a soldier with a specialist military trade within the Royal Army Medical Corps of the British Army and the Royal Air Force.

Role

The fully trained combat medical technician or CMT is capable of:

- assisting with the management of surgical, medical and psychiatric casualties from the onset of the condition until the casualty is admitted to a hospital offering specialist care. This capacity is to include the immediate necessary first aid and other sustaining procedures required to hold a casualty for a limited period in a non-hospital situation

- undertaking the administrative procedures and documentation for casualties in field units, medical reception stations and unit medical centres, including those required for and during casualty

Class 3 and 2 Standards

- Trained in anatomy, physiology and first aid.

- Has a general understanding of medical terminology and is capable of carrying out first aid in an emergency situation until expert medical assistance is available

- Works under supervision to provide assistance to medical officers in field units and medical reception stations

- Assists in setting up field medical units and is trained in medical fieldcraft including the use of radio equipment, navigation by foot or vehicle across country and field medical equipment

- Capable of carrying out basic nursing procedures

- Initiates and maintains casualty documentation and supply/equipment documentation

- Recognises abnormalities in casualty observations, body appearances and consciousness levels

- Trained in basic life support (BLS) to UK Resuscitation Council guidelines

- Trained in Army environmental health issues at unit level

Class 1 Standard

- As for Class 2 and 3, but with additional training and experience

- Provides health advice to non medical junior commanders

- Has a good understanding of anatomy and physiology

- Is able to take control of an emergency situation

- Is trained in basic diagnostic techniques and able to report findings to medical services

- Advises on basic field hygiene

- Capable of advanced first aid and using advanced resuscitation techniques

- Administers non-controlled drugs ordered by a medical officer

- Administers drugs by oral route, inhalations, plus intradermal-, intramuscular- and subcutaneous injection

- Sutures simple wounds

- Maintains, or supervises the maintenance of, and indents for medical equipment

- Trains junior medical assistants

Additionally, at Class 1 the CMT is trained in the procedures and principles of Battlefield Advanced Trauma Life Support (BATLS), which includes advanced life support, cricothyrotomy and thoracentesis.

References

- Vivian Charles McAlister. "Origins of the Canadian School of Surgery" Canadian Journal of Surgery (2007) 50 (5) : 357-363

- Jena, Anupam B.; Sun, Eric C.; Prasad, Vinay (2014). "Does the Declining Lethality of Gunshot Injuries Mask a Rising Epidemic of Gun Violence in the United States?". Journal of General Internal Medicine. 29 (7): 1065–1069. doi:10.1007/s11606-014-2779-z. ISSN 0884-8734. PMC 4061370. PMID 24452421

- "EMERGENCY TREATMENT SECTION : Department of Defense : Free Download & Streaming : Internet Archive". Archive.org. Retrieved 2017-03-28

- Fields, Gary; McWhirter, Cameron (8 December 2012). "In Medical Triumph, Homicides Fall Despite Soaring Gun Violence" – via Wall Street Journal

- Mraz, Steve (17 October 2006). "Last MASH unit becomes Combat Support Hospital, improves capabilities". Stars and Stripes. Retrieved 8 January 2012

- Manring MM, Hawk A, Calhoun JH, Andersen RC (2009). "Treatment of war wounds: a historical review.". Clin Orthop Relat Res. 467 (8): 2168–91. doi:10.1007/s11999-009-0738-5. PMC 2706344. PMID 19219516

Various Medical Emergencies

Medical emergencies are sudden or acute illnesses that can result in long-term injury and even death of a person. Depending on the extent of the injury, it may require different levels of medical attention. The emergencies discussed in this section are head injury, coma, bleeding, wound, cardiac tamponade and stroke. The major categories of medical emergencies are dealt with great details in the chapter.

Medical Emergency

A medical emergency is an acute injury or illness that poses an immediate risk to a person's life or long-term health. These emergencies may require assistance from another person, who should ideally be suitably qualified to do so, although some of these emergencies such as Cardiovascular(Heart), Respiratory, Gastrointestinal cannot be dealt with by the victim themselves. Dependent on the severity of the emergency, and the quality of any treatment given, it may require the involvement of multiple levels of care, from first aiders to Emergency Medical Technicians and emergency physicians.

Any response to an emergency medical situation will depend strongly on the situation, the patient involved and availability of resources to help them. It will also vary depending on whether the emergency occurs whilst in hospital under medical care, or outside of medical care (for instance, in the street or alone at home).

Response

Summoning Emergency Services

For emergencies starting outside of medical care, a key component of providing proper care is to summon the emergency medical services (usually an ambulance), by calling for help using the appropriate local emergency telephone number, such as 999, 911, 111, 112 or 000. After determining that the incident is a medical emergency (as opposed to, for example, a police call), the emergency dispatchers will generally run through a questioning system such as AMPDS in order to assess the priority level of the call, along with the caller's name and location.

First Aid and Assisting Emergency Services

Those who are trained to perform first aid can act within the bounds of the knowledge they have, whilst awaiting the next level of definitive care.

Those who are not able to perform first aid can also assist by remaining calm and staying with the injured or ill person. A common complaint of emergency service personnel is the propensity of people to crowd around the scene of victim, as it is generally unhelpful, making the patient more stressed, and obstructing the smooth working of the emergency services. If possible, first responders should designate a specific person to ensure that the emergency services are called. Another bystander should be sent to wait for their arrival and direct them to the proper location. Additional bystanders can be helpful in ensuring that crowds are moved away from the ill or injured patient, allowing the responder adequate space to work.

Legal Protections for Responders

To prevent the delay of life-saving aid from bystanders, many states of the USA have "Good Samaritan laws" which protect civilian responders who choose to assist in an emergency. In many situations, the general public may delay giving care due to fear of liability should they accidentally cause harm. Good Samaritan laws often protect responders who act within the scope of their knowledge and training, as a "reasonable person" in the same situation would act.

The concept of implied consent can protect first responders in emergency situations. A first responder may not legally touch a patient without the patient's consent. However, consent may be either expressed or implied:

- If a patient is able to make decisions, they must give expressed, informed consent before aid is given.

- However, if a patient is too injured or ill to make decisions - for example, if they are unconscious, have an altered mental status, or cannot communicate - implied consent applies. Implied consent means that treatment can be given, because it is assumed that the patient would want that care.

Usually, once care has begun, a first responder or first aid provider *may not* leave the patient or terminate care until a responder of equal or higher training (such as an emergency medical technician) assumes care. This can constitute abandonment of the patient, and may subject the responder to legal liability. Care must be continued until the patient is transferred to a higher level of care; the situation becomes too unsafe to continue; or the responder is physically unable to continue due to exhaustion or hazards.

Unless the situation is particularly hazardous, and is likely to further endanger the patient, evacuating an injured victim requires special skills, and should be left to the professionals of the emergency medical and fire service.

The Chain of Survival

The principles of the chain of survival apply to medical emergencies where the patient is not breathing and has no pulse. This involves four stages:

1. Early access

2. Early cardiopulmonary resuscitation (CPR)

3. Early defibrillation

4. Early advanced life support (ALS)

Clinical Response

Within hospital settings, an adequate staff is generally present to deal with the average emergency situation. Emergency medicine physicians have training to deal with most medical emergencies, and maintain CPR and Advanced Cardiac Life Support (ACLS) certifications. In disasters or complex emergencies, most hospitals have protocols to summon on-site and off-site staff rapidly.

Both emergency room and inpatient medical emergencies follow the basic protocol of Advanced Cardiac Life Support. Irrespective of the nature of the emergency, adequate blood pressure and oxygenation are required before the cause of the emergency can be eliminated. Possible exceptions include the clamping of arteries in severe hemorrhage.

Non-trauma Emergencies

While the golden hour is a trauma treatment concept, two emergency medical conditions have well-documented time-critical treatment considerations: stroke and myocardial infarction (heart attack). In the case of stroke, there is a window of three hours within which the benefit of thrombolytic drugs outweighs the risk of major bleeding. In the case of a heart attack, rapid stabilization of fatal arrhythmias can prevent sudden cardiac arrest. In addition, there is a direct relationship between time-to-treatment and the success of reperfusion (restoration of blood flow to the heart), including a time-dependent reduction in the mortality and morbidity.

Head Injury

Any injury that results in trauma to the skull or brain can be classified as a head injury. The terms *traumatic brain injury* and *head injury* are often used interchangeably in the medical literature. This broad classification includes neuronal injuries, hemorrhages, vascular injuries, cranial nerve injuries, and subdural hygromas, among many others. These classifications can be further categorized as open (penetrating) or closed head injuries. This depends on if the skull was broken or not. Because head injuries cover such a broad scope of injuries, there are many causes—including accidents, falls, physical assault, or traffic accidents—that can cause head injuries. Many of these are minor, but some can be severe enough to require hospitalization.

The incidence (number of new cases) of head injury is 1.7 million people in the United States alone each year, with about 3% of these incidents leading to death. Adults suffer head injuries more frequently than any age group resulting from falls, motor vehicle crashes, colliding or being struck by an object, or assaults. Children, however, may experience head injuries from accidental falls or intentional causes (such as being struck or shaken) leading to hospitalization.

Unlike a broken bone where trauma to the body is obvious, head trauma can sometimes be conspicuous or inconspicuous. In the case of an open head injury, the skull is cracked and broken by an object that makes contact with the brain. This leads to bleeding. Other obvious symptoms can be neurological in nature. The person may become sleepy, behave abnormally, lose consciousness, vomit, develop a severe headache, have mismatched pupil sizes, and/or be unable to move certain parts of the body. While these symptoms happen right head injury occurs, many problems can develop later in life. Alzheimer's disease, for example, is much more likely to develop in a person who has experienced a head injury.

Classification

Head injuries include both injuries to the brain and those to other parts of the head, such as the scalp and skull. Head injuries can be closed or open. A closed (non-missile) head injury is where the dura mater remains intact. The skull can be fractured, but not necessarily. A penetrating head injury occurs when an object pierces the skull and breaches the dura mater. Brain injuries may be diffuse, occurring over a wide area, or focal, located in a small, specific area. A head injury may cause skull fracture, which may or may not be associated with injury to the brain. Some patients may have linear or depressed skull fractures.If intracranial hemorrhage occurs, a hematoma within the skull can put pressure on the brain. Types of intracranial hemorrage include subdural, subarachnoid, extradural, and intraparenchymal hematoma. Craniotomy surgeries are used in these cases to lessen the pressure by draining off blood.

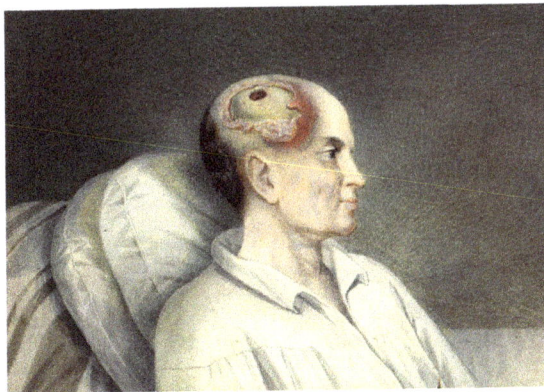

Private Patrick Hughes, Co. K, 4th New York Volunteers, wounded at the Battle of Antietam on September 17, 1862.

Brain injury can occur at the site of impact, but can also be at the opposite side of the skull due to a *contrecoup* effect (the impact to the head can cause the brain to move within the skull, causing the brain to impact the interior of the skull opposite the head-impact). If the impact causes the head to move, the injury may be worsened, because the brain may ricochet inside the skull causing additional impacts, or the brain may stay relatively still (due to inertia) but be hit by the moving skull (both are contrecoup injuries).

- Specific problems after head injury can include

- Skull fracture

- Lacerations to the scalp and resulting hemorrhage of the skin

- Traumatic subdural hematoma, a bleeding below the dura mater which may develop slowly

- Traumatic extradural, or epidural hematoma, bleeding between the dura mater and the skull

- Traumatic subarachnoid hemorrhage

- Cerebral contusion, a bruise of the brain

- Concussion, a loss of function due to trauma

- Dementia pugilistica, or "punch-drunk syndrome", caused by repetitive head injuries, for example in boxing or other contact sports

- A severe injury may lead to a coma or death

- Shaken baby syndrome — a form of child abuse

Concussion

Traumatic brain injury (TBI) is an exchangeable word used for the word concussion. This term refers to a mild brain injury. This injury is a result due to a blow to the head that could make the person's physical, cognitive, and emotional behaviors irregular. Symptoms may include clumsiness, fatigue, confusion, nausea, blurry vision, headaches, and others. Mild concussions are associated with sequelae. Severity is measured using various concussion grading systems.

A slightly greater injury is associated with both anterograde and retrograde amnesia (inability to remember events before or after the injury). The amount of time that the amnesia is present correlates with the severity of the injury. In all cases the patients develop postconcussion syndrome, which includes memory problems, dizziness, tiredness, sickness and depression. Cerebral concussion is the most common head injury seen in children.

Intracranial Hemorrhage

Types of intracranial hemorrhage are roughly grouped into intra-axial and extra-axial. The hemorrhage is considered a focal brain injury; that is, it occurs in a localized spot rather than causing diffuse damage over a wider area.

Intra-axial Hemorrhage

Intra-axial hemorrhage is bleeding within the brain itself, or cerebral hemorrhage. This category includes intraparenchymal hemorrhage, or bleeding within the brain tissue, and intraventricular hemorrhage, bleeding within the brain's ventricles (particularly of premature infants). Intra-axial hemorrhages are more dangerous and harder to treat than extra-axial bleeds.

Extra-axial Hemorrhage

Hematoma type	Epidural	Subdural
Location	Between the skull and the outer endosteal layer of the dura mater	Between the *dura* and the arachnoid
Involved vessel	Temperoparietal locus (most likely) - Middle meningeal artery Frontal locus - anterior ethmoidal artery Occipital locus - transverse or sigmoid sinuses Vertex locus - superior sagittal sinus	Bridging veins
Symptoms(depend on severity)	Lucid interval followed by unconsciousness	Gradually increasing headache and confusion
CT appearance	Biconvex lens	Crescent-shaped

Extra-axial hemorrhage, bleeding that occurs within the skull but outside of the brain tissue, falls into three subtypes:

- Epidural hemorrhage (extradural hemorrhage) which occur between the dura mater (the outermost meninx) and the skull, is caused by trauma. It may result from laceration of an artery, most commonly the middle meningeal artery. This is a very dangerous type of injury because the bleed is from a high-pressure system and deadly increases in intracranial pressure can result rapidly. However, it is the least common type of meningeal bleeding and is seen in 1% to 3% cases of head injury.

    o Patients have a loss of consciousness (LOC), then a lucid interval, then sudden deterioration (vomiting, restlessness, LOC).

    o Head CT shows lenticular (convex) deformity.

- Subdural hemorrhage results from tearing of the bridging veins in the subdural space between the dura and arachnoid mater.

   ◦ Head CT shows crescent-shaped deformity

- Subarachnoid hemorrhage, which occur between the arachnoid and pia menin-geal layers, like intraparenchymal hemorrhage, can result either from trauma or from ruptures of aneurysms or arteriovenous malformations. Blood is seen layering into the brain along sulci and fissures, or filling cisterns (most often the suprasellar cistern because of the presence of the vessels of the circle of Willis and their branchpoints within that space). The classic presentation of subarachnoid hemorrhage is the sudden onset of a severe headache (a thun-derclap headache). This can be a very dangerous entity, and requires emergent neurosurgical evaluation, and sometimes urgent intervention.

Cerebral Contusion

Cerebral contusion is bruising of the brain tissue. The majority of contusions occur in the frontal and temporal lobes. Complications may include cerebral edema and transtentorial herniation. The goal of treatment should be to treat the increased intra-cranial pressure. The prognosis is guarded.

Diffuse Axonal Injury

Diffuse axonal injury, or DAI, usually occurs as the result of an acceleration or deceler-ation motion, not necessarily an impact. Axons are stretched and damaged when parts of the brain of differing density slide over one another. Prognoses vary widely depend-ing on the extent of damage.

Signs and Symptoms

Presentation varies according to the injury. Some patients with head trauma stabi-lize and other patients deteriorate. A patient may present with or without neurologi-cal deficit. Patients with concussion may have a history of seconds to minutes uncon-sciousness, then normal arousal. Disturbance of vision and equilibrium may also occur. Common symptoms of head injury include coma, confusion, drowsiness, personality change, seizures, nausea and vomiting, headache and a lucid interval, during which a patient appears conscious only to deteriorate later.

Symptoms of skull fracture can include:

- leaking cerebrospinal fluid (a clear fluid drainage from nose, mouth or ear) may be and is strongly indicative of basilar skull fracture and the tearing of sheaths surrounding the brain, which can lead to secondary brain infection.

- visible deformity or depression in the head or face; for example a sunken eye can indicate a maxillar fracture

- an eye that cannot move or is deviated to one side can indicate that a broken facial bone is pinching a nerve that innervates eye muscles

- wounds or bruises on the scalp or face.

- Basilar skull fractures, those that occur at the base of the skull, are associated with Battle's sign, a subcutaneous bleed over the mastoid, hemotympanum, and cerebrospinal fluid rhinorrhea and otorrhea.

Because brain injuries can be life-threatening, even people with apparently slight injuries, with no noticeable signs or complaints, require close observation; They have a chance for severe symptoms later on. The caretakers of those patients with mild trauma who are released from the hospital are frequently advised to rouse the patient several times during the next 12 to 24 hours to assess for worsening symptoms.

The Glasgow Coma Scale (GCS) is a tool for measuring degree of unconsciousness and is thus a useful tool for determining severity of injury. The Pediatric Glasgow Coma Scale is used in young children. The widely used PECARN Pediatric Head Injury/Trauma Algorithm helps physicians weigh risk-benefit of imaging in a clinical setting given multiple factors about the patient - including mechanism/location of injury, age of patient, and GCS score.

Causes

Common causes of head injury are motor vehicle traffic collisions, home and occupational accidents, falls, and assaults. Wilson's disease has also been indicative of head injury. According to the United States CDC, 32% of traumatic brain injuries (another, more specific, term for head injuries) are caused by falls, 10% by assaults, 16.5% by being struck or against something, 17% by motor vehicle accidents, 21% by other/unknown ways. In addition, the highest rate of injury is among children ages 0–14 and adults age 65 and older.

Diagnosis

The need for imaging in patients who have suffered a minor head injury is debated. A non-contrast CT of the head should be performed immediately in all those who have suffered a moderate or severe head injury,an MRI is also an option. Computed tomography (CT) has become the diagnostic modality of choice for head trauma due to its accuracy, reliability, safety, and wide availability. The changes in microcirculation, impaired auto-regulation, cerebral edema, and axonal injury start as soon as head injury occurs and manifest as clinical, biochemical, and radiological changes.

Management

Most head injuries are of a benign nature and require no treatment beyond analgesics and close monitoring for potential complications such as intracranial bleeding. If the brain has been severely damaged by trauma, neurosurgical evaluation may be useful. Treatments may involve controlling elevated intracranial pressure. This can include sedation, paralytics, cerebrospinal fluid diversion. Second line alternatives include decompressive craniectomy (Jagannathan et al. found a net 65% favorable outcomes rate in pediatric patients), barbiturate coma, hypertonic saline and hypothermia. Although all of these methods have potential benefits, there has been no randomized study that has shown unequivocal benefit.

Clinicians will often consult clinical decision support rules such as the Canadian CT Head Rule or the New Orleans/Charity Head injury/Trauma Rule to decide if the patient needs further imaging studies or observation only. Rules like these are usually studied in depth by multiple research groups with large patient cohorts to ensure accuracy given the risk of adverse events in this area.

Prognosis

In children with uncomplicated minor head injuries the risk of intra cranial bleeding over the next year is rare at 2 cases per 1 million. In some cases transient neurological disturbances may occur, lasting minutes to hours. Malignant post traumatic cerebral swelling can develop unexpectedly in stable patients after an injury, as can post traumatic seizures. Recovery in children with neurologic deficits will vary. Children with neurologic deficits who improve daily are more likely to recover, while those who are vegetative for months are less likely to improve. Most patients without deficits have full recovery. However, persons who sustain head trauma resulting in unconsciousness for an hour or more have twice the risk of developing Alzheimer's disease later in life.

Head injury may be associated with a neck injury. Bruises on the back or neck, neck pain, or pain radiating to the arms are signs of cervical spine injury and merit spinal immobilization via application of a cervical collar and possibly a long board.If the neurological exam is normal this is reassuring. Reassessment is needed if there is a worsening headache, seizure, one sided weakness, or has persistent vomiting.

To combat overuse of Head CT Scans yielding negative intracranial hemorrhage, which unnecessarily expose patients to radiation and increase time in the hospital and cost of the visit, multiple clinical decision support rules have been developed to help clinicians weigh the option to scan a patient with a head injury. Among these are the Canadian Head CT rule, the PECARN Head Injury/Trauma Algorithm, and the New Orleans/Charity Head Injury/Trauma Rule all help clinicians make these decisions using easily obtained information and noninvasive practices.

Coma

Coma is a state of unconsciousness in which a person cannot be awakened; fails to respond normally to painful stimuli, light, or sound; lacks a normal wake-sleep cycle;

and does not initiate voluntary actions. A person in a state of coma is described as being *comatose*. A distinction is made in the medical community between a coma and a medically induced coma, the former is a result of circumstances beyond the control of the medical community, while the latter is a means by which medical professionals may allow a patient's injuries to heal in a controlled environment.

A comatose person exhibits a complete absence of wakefulness and is unable to consciously feel, speak, hear, or move. For a patient to maintain consciousness, two important neurological components must function. The first is the cerebral cortex—the gray matter that forms the outer layer of the brain. The other is a structure located in the brainstem, called reticular activating system (RAS). Injury to either or both of these components is sufficient to cause a patient to experience a coma. The cerebral cortex is a group of tight, dense, "gray matter" composed of the nuclei of the neurons whose axons then form the "white matter," and is responsible for perception, relay of the sensory input via the thalamic pathway, and many other neurological functions, including complex thinking.

RAS, on the other hand, is a more primitive structure in the brainstem which includes the reticular formation (RF). The RAS area of the brain has two tracts, the ascending and descending tract. Made up of a system of acetylcholine-producing neurons, the ascending track, or ascending reticular activating system (ARAS), works to arouse and wake up the brain, from the RF, through the thalamus, and then finally to the cerebral cortex. A failure in ARAS functioning may then lead to a coma. The word is from the Greek *koma*, meaning "deep sleep."

Signs and Symptoms

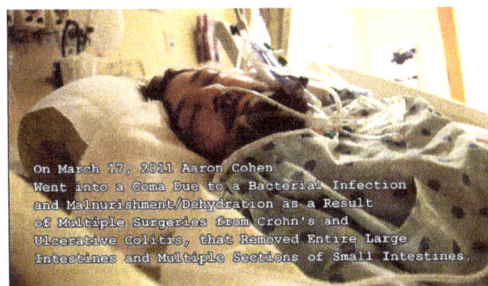

On March 17, 2011 Aaron Cohen
Went into a Coma Due to a Bacterial Infection
and Malnurishment/Dehydration as a Result
of Multiple Surgeries from Crohn's and
Ulcerative Colitis, that Removed Entire Large
Intestines and Multiple Sections of Small Intestines.

Image of a man in a coma.

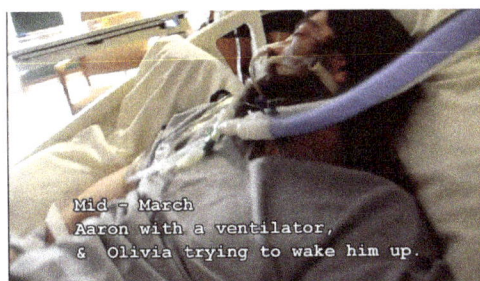

Mid - March
Aaron with a ventilator,
& Olivia trying to wake him up.

Image of the man still unresponsive to stimuli.

Generally, a person who is unable to voluntarily open the eyes, does not have a sleep-wake cycle, is unresponsive in spite of strong tactile (painful) or verbal stimuli, and who generally scores between 3 and 8 on the Glasgow Coma Scale is considered in a coma. Coma may have developed in humans as a response to injury to allow the body to pause bodily actions and heal the most immediate injuries before waking. It therefore could be a compensatory state in which the body's expenditure of energy is not superfluous. The severity and mode of onset of coma depends on the underlying cause. For instance, severe hypoglycemia (low blood sugar) or hypercapnia (increased carbon dioxide levels in the blood) initially cause mild agitation and confusion, but progress to obtundation, stupor, and finally, complete unconsciousness. In contrast, coma resulting from a severe traumatic brain injury or subarachnoid hemorrhage can be instantaneous. The mode of onset may therefore be indicative of the underlying cause.

Causes of Coma

Coma may result from a variety of conditions, including intoxication (such as drug abuse, overdose or misuse of over the counter medications, prescribed medication, or controlled substances), metabolic abnormalities, central nervous system diseases, acute neurologic injuries such as strokes or herniations, hypoxia, hypothermia, hypoglycemia, Eclampsia or traumatic injuries such as head trauma caused by falls, drowning accidents, or vehicle collisions. It may also be deliberately induced by pharmaceutical agents during major neurosurgery, to preserve higher brain functions following brain trauma, or to save the patient from extreme pain during healing of injuries or diseases.

Forty percent of comatose states result from drug poisoning. Drugs damage or weaken the synaptic functioning in the ARAS and keep the system from properly functioning to arouse the brain. Secondary effects of drugs, which include abnormal heart rate and blood pressure, as well as abnormal breathing and sweating, may also indirectly harm the functioning of the ARAS and lead to a coma. Seizures and hallucinations have shown to also play a major role in ARAS malfunction. Given that drug poisoning is the cause for a large portion of patients in a coma, hospitals first test all comatose patients by observing pupil size and eye movement, through the vestibular-ocular reflex.

The second most common cause of coma, which makes up about 25% of comatose patients, occurs from lack of oxygen, generally resulting from cardiac arrest. The Central Nervous System (CNS) requires a great deal of oxygen for its neurons. Oxygen deprivation in the brain, also known as hypoxia, causes neuronal extracellular sodium and calcium to decrease and intracellular calcium to increase, which harms neuron communication. Lack of oxygen in the brain also causes ATP exhaustion and cellular breakdown from cytoskeleton damage and nitric oxide production.

Twenty percent of comatose states result from the side effects of a stroke. During a stroke, blood flow to part of the brain is restricted or blocked. An ischemic stroke, brain hemorrhage, or tumor may cause such cessation of blood flow. Lack of blood to cells in the brain prevents oxygen from getting to the neurons, and consequently causes cells to become disrupted and eventually die. As brain cells die, brain tissue continues to deteriorate, which may affect functioning of the ARAS.

The remaining 15% of comatose cases result from trauma, excessive blood loss, malnutrition, hypothermia, hyperthermia, abnormal glucose levels, and many other biological disorders.

Diagnosis

Diagnosis of coma is simple, but diagnosing the cause of the underlying disease process is often challenging. The first priority in treatment of a comatose patient is stabilization following the basic ABCs (standing for airway, breathing, and circulation). Once a person in a coma is stable, investigations are performed to assess the underlying cause. Investigative methods are divided into physical examination findings and imaging (such as CAT scan, MRI, etc.) and special studies (EEG, etc.)

Diagnostic Steps

When an unconscious patient enters a hospital, the hospital utilizes a series of diagnostic steps to identify the cause of unconsciousness. According to Young, the following steps should be taken when dealing with a patient possibly in a coma:

1. Perform a general examination and medical history check

2. Make sure the patient is in an actual comatose state and or is not in locked-in state (patient is either able to voluntarily move their eyes or blink) or psychogenic unresponsiveness (caloric stimulation of the vestibular apparatus results in slow deviation of eyes towards the stimulation followed by rapid correction to mid-line. This response cannot be voluntarily suppressed, so if the patient does not have this response, psychogenic coma can be ruled out.)

3. Find the site of the brain that may be causing coma (i.e., brain stem, back of brain...) and assess the severity of the coma with the Glasgow coma scale

4. Take blood work to see if drugs were involved or if it was a result of hypoventilation/hyperventilation

5. Check for levels of "serum glucose, calcium, sodium, potassium, magnesium, phosphate, urea, and creatinine"

6. Perform brain scans to observe any abnormal brain functioning using either CT or MRI scans

7. Continue to monitor brain waves and identify seizures of patient using EEGs

Initial Assessment and Evaluation

In the initial assessment of coma, it is common to gauge the level of consciousness by spontaneously exhibited actions, response to vocal stimuli ("Can you hear me?"), and painful stimuli; this is known as the AVPU (alert, vocal stimuli, painful stimuli, unresponsive) scale. More elaborate scales, such as the Glasgow Coma Scale, quantify an individual's reactions such as eye opening, movement and verbal response on a scale; Glasgow Coma Scale (GCS) is an indication of the extent of brain injury varying from 3 (indicating severe brain injury and death) to a maximum of 15 (indicating mild or no brain injury).

In those with deep unconsciousness, there is a risk of asphyxiation as the control over the muscles in the face and throat is diminished. As a result, those presenting to a hospital with coma are typically assessed for this risk ("airway management"). If the risk of asphyxiation is deemed high, doctors may use various devices (such as an oropharyngeal airway, nasopharyngeal airway or endotracheal tube) to safeguard the airway.

Physical Examination Findings

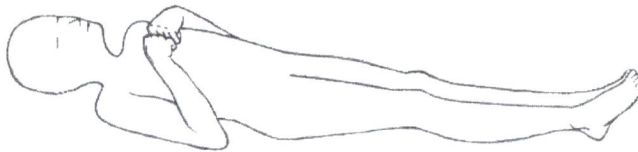

Decorticate posturing, indicating a lesion at the red nucleus or above. This positioning is stereotypical for upper brain stem, or cortical damage. The other variant is decerebrate posturing, not seen in this picture.

Physical examination is critical after stabilization. It should include vital signs, a general portion dedicated to making observations about the patient's respiration (breathing pattern), body movements (if any), and of the patient's body habitus (physique); it should also include assessment of the brainstem and cortical function through special reflex tests such as the oculocephalic reflex test (doll's eyes test), oculovestibular reflex test (cold caloric test), nasal tickle, corneal reflex, and the gag reflex.

Vital signs in medicine are temperature (rectal is most accurate), blood pressure, heart rate (pulse), respiratory rate, and oxygen saturation. It should be easy to evaluate these vitals quickly to gain insight into a patient's metabolism, fluid status, heart function, vascular integrity, and tissue oxygenation.

Respiratory pattern (breathing rhythm) is significant and should be noted in a comatose patient. Certain stereotypical patterns of breathing have been identified including Cheyne–Stokes, a form of breathing in which the patient's breathing pattern is described as alternating episodes of hyperventilation and apnea. This is a dangerous pattern and is often seen in pending herniations, extensive cortical lesions, or brainstem damage. Another pattern of breathing is apneustic breathing, which is characterized by sudden pauses of inspiration and is due to a lesion of the pons. Ataxic breathing is irregular and is due to a lesion (damage) of the medulla.

Assessment of posture and body habitus is the next step. It involves general observation about the patient's positioning. There are often two stereotypical postures seen in comatose patients. Decorticate posturing is a stereotypical posturing in which the patient has arms flexed at the elbow, and arms adducted toward the body, with both legs extended. Decerebrate posturing is a stereotypical posturing in which the legs are similarly extended (stretched), but the arms are also stretched (extended at the elbow). The posturing is critical since it indicates where the damage is in the central nervous system. A decorticate posturing indicates a lesion (a point of damage) at or above the red nucleus, whereas a decerebrate posturing indicates a lesion at or below the red nucleus. In other words, a decorticate lesion is closer to the cortex, as opposed to a decerebrate cortex that is closer to the brainstem.

Oculocephalic reflex also known as the doll's eye is performed to assess the integrity of the brainstem. Patient's eyelids are gently elevated and the cornea is visualized. The patient's head is then moved to the patient's left, to observe if the eyes stay or deviate toward the patient's right; same maneuver is attempted on the opposite side. If the patient's eyes move in a direction opposite to the direction of the rotation of the head, then the patient is said to have an intact brainstem. However, failure of both eyes to move to one side, can indicate damage or destruction of the affected side. In special cases, where only one eye deviates and the other does not, this often indicates a lesion (or damage) of the medial longitudinal fasciculus (MLF), which is a brainstem nerve tract. Caloric reflex test also evaluates both cortical and brainstem function; cold water is injected into one ear and the patient is observed for eye movement; if the patient's eyes slowly deviate toward the ear where the water was injected, then the brainstem is intact, however failure to deviate toward the injected ear indicates damage of the brainstem on that side. Cortex is responsible for a rapid nystagmus away from this deviated position and is often seen in patients who are conscious or merely lethargic.

An important part of the physical exam is also assessment of the cranial nerves. Due to the unconscious status of the patient, only a limited number of the nerves can be assessed. These include the cranial nerves number 2 (CN II), number 3 (CN III), number 5 (CN V), number 7 (CN VII), and cranial nerves 9 and 10 (CN IX, CN X). Gag reflex helps assess cranial nerves 9 and 10. Pupil reaction to light is important because it shows an intact retina, and cranial nerve number 2 (CN II); if pupils are reactive to light, then that also indicates that the cranial nerve number 3 (CN III) (or at least its parasympathetic fibers) are intact. Corneal reflex assess the integrity of cranial nerve number 7 (CN VII), and cranial nerve number 5 (CN V). Cranial nerve number 5 (CN V), and its ophthalmic branch (V_1) are responsible for the afferent arm of the reflex, and the cranial nerve number 7 (CN VII) also known a facial nerve, is responsible for the efferent arm, causing contraction of the muscle orbicularis oculi resulting in closing of the eyes.

Pupil assessment is often a critical portion of a comatose examination, as it can give information as to the cause of the coma; the following table is a technical, medical guideline for common pupil findings and their possible interpretations:

Pupil sizes (left eye vs. right eye)	Possible interpretation
	Normal eye with two pupils equal in size and reactive to light. This means that the patient is probably not in a coma and is probably lethargic, under influence of a drug, or sleeping.
	"Pinpoint" pupils indicate heroin or opiate overdose, and can be responsible for a patient's coma. The pinpoint pupils are still reactive to light, bilaterally (in both eyes, not just one). Another possibility is the damage of the pons.
	One pupil is dilated and unreactive, while the other is normal (in this case, the right eye is dilated, while the left eye is normal in size). This could mean a damage to the oculomotor nerve (cranial nerve number 3, CN III) on the right side, or possibility of vascular involvement.
	Both pupils are dilated and unreactive to light. This could be due to overdose of certain medications, hypothermia or severe anoxia (lack of oxygen).

Imaging and Special Tests Findings

Imaging basically encompasses computed tomography (CAT or CT) scan of the brain, or MRI for example, and is performed to identify specific causes of the coma, such as hemorrhage in the brain or herniation of the brain structures. Special tests such as an EEG can also show a lot about the activity level of the cortex such as semantic processing, presence of seizures, and are important available tools not only for the assessment of the cortical activity but also for predicting the likelihood of the patient's awakening. The autonomous responses such as the skin conductance response may also provide further insight on the patient's emotional processing.

History

When diagnosing any neurological condition, history and examination are fundamental. History is obtained by family, friends or EMS. The Glasgow Coma Scale is a helpful system used to examine and determine the depth of coma, track patients progress and predict outcome as best as possible. In general a correct diagnosis can be achieved by combining findings from physical exam, imaging, and history components and directs the appropriate therapy.

Severity and Classification

A coma can be classified as (1) supratentorial (above Tentorium cerebelli), (2) infratentorial (below Tentorium cerebelli), (3) metabolic or (4) diffused. This classification is merely dependent on the position of the original damage that caused the coma, and does not correlate with severity or the prognosis. The severity of coma impairment however is categorized into several levels. Patients may or may not progress through these levels. In the first level, the brain responsiveness lessens, normal reflexes are lost, the patient no longer responds to pain and cannot hear.

The Rancho Los Amigos Scale is a complex scale that has eight separate levels, and is often used in the first few weeks or months of coma while the patient is under closer observation, and when shifts between levels are more frequent.

Treatment

Medical Treatment

The treatment hospitals use on comatose patients depends on both the severity and cause of the comatose state. Although the best treatment for comatose patients remains unknown, hospitals usually place comatose patients in an Intensive Care Unit (ICU) immediately. In the ICU, the hospital monitors a patient's breathing and brain activity through CT scans. Attention must first be directed to maintaining the patient's respiration and circulation, using intubation and ventilation, administration of intravenous fluids or blood and other supportive care as needed. Once a patient is stable and no longer in immediate danger, the medical staff may concentrate on maintaining the health of patient's physical state. The concentration is directed to preventing infections such as pneumonias, bedsores (decubitus ulcers), and providing balanced nutrition. Infections may appear from the patient not being able to move around, and being confined to the bed. The nursing staff moves the patient every 2–3 hours from side to side and depending on the state of consciousness sometimes to a chair. The goal is to move the patient as much as possible to try to avoid bedsores, atelectasis and pneumonia. Pneumonia can occur from the person's inability to swallow leading to aspiration, lack of gag reflex or from feeding tube, (aspiration pneumonia). Physical therapy may also be used to prevent contractures and orthopedic deformities that would limit recovery for those patients who awaken from coma.

A person in a coma may become restless, or seize and need special care to prevent them from hurting themselves. Medicine may be given to calm such individuals. Patients who are restless may also try to pull on tubes or dressings so soft cloth wrist restraints may be put on. Side rails on the bed should be kept up to prevent the patient from falling.

Methods to wake comatose patients include reversing the cause of the coma (i.e., glucose shock if low sugar), giving medication to stop brain swelling, or inducing hypothermia. Inducing hypothermia on comatose patients provides one of the main treatments for patients after suffering from cardiac arrest. In this treatment, medical personnel expose patients to "external or intravascular cooling" at 32-34 °C for 24 hours; this treatment cools patients down about 2-3 °C less than normal body temperature. In 2002, Baldursdottir and her coworkers found that in the hospital, more comatose patients survived after induced hypothermia than patients that remained at normal body temperature. For this reason, the hospital chose to continue the induced hypothermia technique for all of its comatose patients that suffered from cardiac arrest.

Emotional Challenges

Coma has a wide variety of emotional reactions from the family members of the affected patients, as well as the primary care givers taking care of the patients. Common reactions, such as desperation, anger, frustration, and denial are possible. The focus of the patient care should be on creating an amicable relationship with the family members or dependents of a comatose patient as well as creating a rapport with the medical staff.

Prognosis

Comas can last from several days to several weeks. In more severe cases a coma may last for over five weeks, while some have lasted as long as several years. After this time, some patients gradually come out of the coma, some progress to a vegetative state, and others die. Some patients who have entered a vegetative state go on to regain a degree of awareness. Others remain in a vegetative state for years or even decades (the longest recorded period being 42 years).

The outcome for coma and vegetative state depends on the cause, location, severity and extent of neurological damage. A deeper coma alone does not necessarily mean a slimmer chance of recovery, because some people in deep coma recover well while others in a so-called milder coma sometimes fail to improve.

People may emerge from a coma with a combination of physical, intellectual, and psychological difficulties that need special attention. Recovery usually occurs gradually—patients acquire more and more ability to respond. Some patients never progress beyond very basic responses, but many recover full awareness. Regaining consciousness is not instant: in the first days, patients are only awake for a few minutes, and duration of time awake gradually increases. This is unlike the situation in many movies where people who awake from comas are instantly able to continue their normal lives. In reality, the coma patient awakes sometimes in a profound state of confusion, not knowing how they got there and sometimes suffering from dysarthria, the inability to articulate any speech, and with many other disabilities.

Predicted chances of recovery are variable owing to different techniques used to measure the extent of neurological damage. All the predictions are based on statistical rates with some level of chance for recovery present: a person with a low chance of recovery may still awaken. Time is the best general predictor of a chance of recovery: after four months of coma caused by brain damage, the chance of partial recovery is less than 15%, and the chance of full recovery is very low.

The most common cause of death for a person in a vegetative state is secondary infection such as pneumonia, which can occur in patients who lie still for extended periods.

There are reports of patients coming out of coma after long periods of time. After 19 years in a minimally conscious state, Terry Wallis spontaneously began speaking and regained awareness of his surroundings.

A brain-damaged man, trapped in a coma-like state for six years, was brought back to consciousness in 2003 by doctors who planted electrodes deep inside his brain. The method, called deep brain stimulation (DBS) successfully roused communication, complex movement and eating ability in the 38-year-old American man who suffered a traumatic brain injury. His injuries left him in a minimally conscious state (MCS), a condition akin to a coma but characterized by occasional, but brief, evidence of environmental and self-awareness that coma patients lack.

Comas lasting seconds to minutes result in post-traumatic amnesia (PTA) that lasts hours to days; recovery plateau occurs over days to weeks. Comas that last hours to days result in PTA lasting days to weeks; recovery plateau occurs over months. Comas lasting weeks result in PTA that lasts months; recovery plateau occurs over months to years.

Society and Culture

Research by Dr. Eelco Wijdicks on the depiction of comas in movies was published in Neurology in May 2006. Dr. Wijdicks studied 30 films (made between 1970 and 2004) that portrayed actors in prolonged comas, and he concluded that only two films accurately depicted the state of a coma victim and the agony of waiting for a patient to awaken: *Reversal of Fortune* (1990) and *The Dreamlife of Angels* (1998). The remaining 28 were criticized for portraying miraculous awakenings with no lasting side effects, unrealistic depictions of treatments and equipment required, and comatose patients remaining muscular and tanned.

Bleeding

Bleeding, also known as hemorrhaging or haemorrhaging, is blood escaping from the circulatory system. Bleeding can occur internally, where blood leaks from blood vessels inside the body, or externally, either through a natural opening such as the mouth, nose, ear, urethra, vagina or anus, or through a break in the skin. Hypovolemia is a massive decrease in blood volume, and death by excessive loss of blood is referred to as exsanguination. Typically, a healthy person can endure a loss of 10–15% of the total blood volume without serious medical difficulties (by comparison, blood donation typically takes 8–10% of the donor's blood volume). The stopping or controlling of bleeding is called hemostasis and is an important part of both first aid and surgery. The use of "super glue" to prevent bleeding and seal battle wound was designed and first used in the Vietnam War. Today many medical treatments use a medical version of "super glue" instead of using traditional stitches used for small wounds that need to be closed at the skin level.

Classification

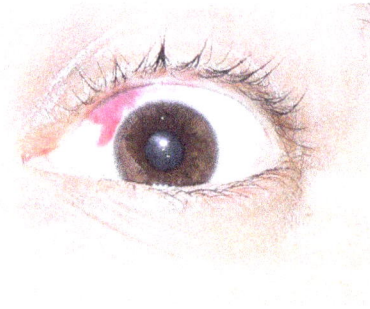

A subconjunctival hemorrhage is a common and relatively minor post-LASIK complication.

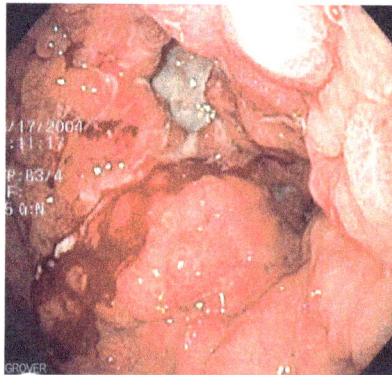

The endoscopic image of linitis plastica, a type of stomach cancer leading to a leather bottle-like appearance with blood coming out of it.

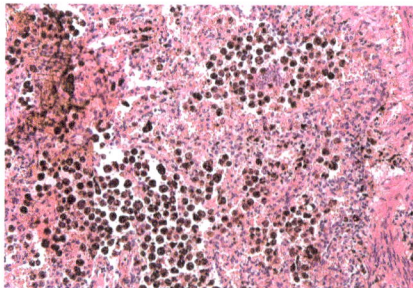

Micrograph showing abundant hemosiderin-laden alveolar macrophages (dark brown), as seen in a pulmonary hemorrhage. H&E stain.

Blood Loss

Hemorrhaging is broken down into four classes by the American College of Surgeons' advanced trauma life support (ATLS).

- Class I Hemorrhage involves up to 15% of blood volume. There is typically no change in vital signs and fluid resuscitation is not usually necessary.

- Class II Hemorrhage involves 15-30% of total blood volume. A patient is often tachycardic (rapid heart beat) with a narrowing of the difference between the systolic and diastolic blood pressures. The body attempts to compensate with peripheral vasoconstriction. Skin may start to look pale and be cool to the touch. The patient may exhibit slight changes in behavior. Volume resuscitation with crystalloids (Saline solution or Lactated Ringer's solution) is all that is typically required. Blood transfusion is not typically required.

- Class III Hemorrhage involves loss of 30-40% of circulating blood volume. The patient's blood pressure drops, the heart rate increases, peripheral hypoperfusion (shock), such as capillary refill worsens, and the mental status worsens. Fluid resuscitation with crystalloid and blood transfusion are usually necessary.

- Class IV Hemorrhage involves loss of >40% of circulating blood volume. The limit of the body's compensation is reached and aggressive resuscitation is required to prevent death.

This system is basically the same as used in the staging of hypovolemic shock.

Individuals in excellent physical and cardiovascular shape may have more effective compensatory mechanisms before experiencing cardiovascular collapse. These patients may look deceptively stable, with minimal derangements in vital signs, while having poor peripheral perfusion. Elderly patients or those with chronic medical conditions may have less tolerance to blood loss, less ability to compensate, and may take medications such as betablockers that can potentially blunt the cardiovascular response. Care must be taken in the assessment.

Massive Hemorrhage

Definitions vary. One definition used is the need for more than 3 to 5 units of packed red blood cells in a day.

World Health Organization

The World Health Organization made a standardized grading scale to measure the severity of bleeding.

Grade 0	no bleeding
Grade 1	petechial bleeding;
Grade 2	mild blood loss (clinically significant);
Grade 3	gross blood loss, requires transfusion (severe);
Grade 4	debilitating blood loss, retinal or cerebral associated with fatality

Types

- Mouth

  - Tooth eruption – losing a tooth

  - Hematemesis – vomiting fresh blood

  - Hemoptysis – coughing up blood from the lungs

- Anus

  - Melena - upper gastrointestinal bleeding

  - Hematochezia – lower gastrointestinal bleeding, or brisk upper gastrointestinal bleeding

- Urinary tract

  - Hematuria – blood in the urine from urinary bleeding

- Upper head

  - Intracranial hemorrhage – bleeding in the skull.

  - Cerebral hemorrhage – a type of intracranial hemorrhage, bleeding within the brain tissue itself.

  - Intracerebral hemorrhage – bleeding in the brain caused by the rupture of a blood vessel within the head.

  - Subarachnoid hemorrhage (SAH) implies the presence of blood within the subarachnoid space from some pathologic process. The common medical use of the term SAH refers to the nontraumatic types of hemorrhages, usually from rupture of a berry aneurysm or arteriovenous malformation(AVM).

- Lungs

  - Pulmonary hemorrhage

- Gynecologic

  o Vaginal bleeding

    ▪ Postpartum hemorrhage

    ▪ Breakthrough bleeding

  o *Ovarian bleeding.* This is a potentially catastrophic and not so rare complication among lean patients with polycystic ovary syndrome undergoing transvaginal oocyte retrieval.

- Gastrointestinal

  o Upper gastrointestinal bleed

  o Lower gastrointestinal bleed

  o Occult gastrointestinal bleed

Causes

Bleeding arises due to either traumatic injury, underlying medical condition, or a combination.

Traumatic Injury

Traumatic bleeding is caused by some type of injury. There are different types of wounds which may cause traumatic bleeding. These include:

- Abrasion - Also called a graze, this is caused by transverse action of a foreign object against the skin, and usually does not penetrate below the epidermis

- Excoriation - In common with Abrasion, this is caused by mechanical destruction of the skin, although it usually has an underlying medical cause

- Hematoma - Caused by damage to a blood vessel that in turn causes blood to collect under the skin.

- Laceration - Irregular wound caused by blunt impact to soft tissue overlying hard tissue or tearing such as in childbirth. In some instances, this can also be used to describe an incision.

- Incision - A cut into a body tissue or organ, such as by a scalpel, made during surgery.

- Puncture Wound - Caused by an object that penetrated the skin and underlying layers, such as a nail, needle or knife.

- Contusion - Also known as a bruise, this is a blunt trauma damaging tissue under the surface of the skin

- Crushing Injuries - Caused by a great or extreme amount of force applied over a period of time. The extent of a crushing injury may not immediately present itself.

- Ballistic Trauma - Caused by a projectile weapon such as a firearm. This may include two external wounds (entry and exit) and a contiguous wound between the two.

The pattern of injury, evaluation and treatment will vary with the mechanism of the injury. Blunt trauma causes injury via a shock effect; delivering energy over an area. Wounds are often not straight and unbroken skin may hide significant injury. Penetrating trauma follows the course of the injurious device. As the energy is applied in a more focused fashion, it requires less energy to cause significant injury. Any body organ, including bone and brain, can be injured and bleed. Bleeding may not be readily apparent; internal organs such as the liver, kidney and spleen may bleed into the abdominal cavity. The only apparent signs may come with blood loss. Bleeding from a bodily orifice, such as the rectum, nose, or ears may signal internal bleeding, but cannot be relied upon. Bleeding from a medical procedure also falls into this category.

Medical Condition

"Medical bleeding" denotes hemorrhage as a result of an underlying medical condition (i.e. causes of bleeding that are not directly due to trauma). Blood can escape from blood vessels as a result of 3 basic patterns of injury:

- Intravascular changes - changes of the blood within vessels (e.g. ↑ blood pressure, ↓ clotting factors)

- Intramural changes - changes arising within the walls of blood vessels (e.g. aneurysms, dissections, AVMs, vasculitides)

- Extravascular changes - changes arising outside blood vessels (e.g. *H pylori* infection, brain abscess, brain tumor)

The underlying scientific basis for blood clotting and hemostasis is discussed in detail. The discussion here is limited to the common practical aspects of blood clot formation which manifest as bleeding.

Some medical conditions can also make patients susceptible to bleeding. These are conditions that affect the normal hemostatic (bleeding-control) functions of the body. Such conditions either are, or cause, bleeding diatheses. Hemostasis involves several components. The main components of the hemostatic system include platelets and the coagulation system.

Platelets are small blood components that form a plug in the blood vessel wall that stops bleeding. Platelets also produce a variety of substances that stimulate the production of a blood clot. One of the most common causes of increased bleeding risk is exposure to non-steroidal anti-inflammatory drugs (or "NSAIDs"). The prototype for these drugs is aspirin, which inhibits the production of thromboxane. NSAIDs inhibit the activation of platelets, and thereby increase the risk of bleeding. The effect of aspirin is irreversible; therefore, the inhibitory effect of aspirin is present until the platelets have been replaced (about ten days). Other NSAIDs, such as "ibuprofen" (Motrin) and related drugs, are reversible and therefore, the effect on platelets is not as long-lived.

There are several named coagulation factors that interact in a complex way to form blood clots as discussed. Deficiencies of coagulation factors are associated with clinical bleeding. For instance, deficiency of Factor VIII causes classic Hemophilia A while deficiencies of Factor IX cause "Christmas disease"(hemophilia B). Antibodies to Factor VIII can also inactivate the Factor VII and precipitate bleeding that is very difficult to control. This is a rare condition that is most likely to occur in older patients and in those with autoimmune diseases. von Willebrand disease is another common bleeding disorder. It is caused by a deficiency of or abnormal function of the "von Willebrand" factor, which is involved in platelet activation. Deficiencies in other factors, such as factor XIII or factor VII are occasionally seen, but may not be associated with severe bleeding and are not as commonly diagnosed.

In addition to NSAID-related bleeding, another common cause of bleeding is that related to the medication, warfarin ("Coumadin" and others). This medication needs to be closely monitored as the bleeding risk can be markedly increased by interactions with other medications. Warfarin acts by inhibiting the production of Vitamin K in the gut. Vitamin K is required for the production of the clotting factors, II, VII, IX, and X in the liver. One of the most common causes of warfarin-related bleeding is taking antibiotics. The gut bacteria make vitamin K and are killed by antibiotics. This decreases vitamin K levels and therefore the production of these clotting factors.

Deficiencies of platelet function may require platelet transfusion while deficiencies of clotting factors may require transfusion of either fresh frozen plasma or specific clotting factors, such as Factor VIII for patients with hemophilia.

Imaging

Dioxaborolane chemistry enables radioactive fluoride (^{18}F) labeling of red blood cells, which allows for positron emission tomography (PET) imaging of intracerebral hemorrhages.

Wound

A wound is a type of injury which happens relatively quickly in which skin is torn, cut, or punctured (an *open* wound), or where blunt force trauma causes a contusion (a *closed* wound). In pathology, it specifically refers to a sharp injury which damages the dermis of the skin.

Classification

According to level of contamination, a wound can be classified as:

- Clean wound – made under sterile conditions where there are no organisms present, and the skin is likely to heal without complications.

- Contaminated wound – usually resulting from accidental injury; there are pathogenic organisms and foreign bodies in the wound.

- Infected wound – the wound has pathogenic organisms present and multiplying, exhibiting clinical signs of infection (yellow appearance, soreness, redness, oozing pus).

- Colonized wound – a chronic situation, containing pathogenic organisms, difficult to heal (i.e. bedsore).

Open

Open wounds can be classified according to the object that caused the wound:

- Incisions or incised wounds – caused by a clean, sharp-edged object such as a knife, razor, or glass splinter.

- Lacerations – irregular tear-like wounds caused by some blunt trauma. Lacerations and incisions may appear linear (regular) or stellate (irregular). The term *laceration* is commonly misused in reference to incisions.

- Abrasions (grazes) – superficial wounds in which the topmost layer of the skin (the epidermis) is scraped off. Abrasions are often caused by a sliding fall onto a rough surface.

- Avulsions – injuries in which a body structure is forcibly detached from its normal point of insertion. A type of amputation where the extremity is pulled off rather than cut off.

- Puncture wounds – caused by an object puncturing the skin, such as a splinter, nail or needle.

- Penetration wounds – caused by an object such as a knife entering and coming out from the skin.

- Gunshot wounds – caused by a bullet or similar projectile driving into or through the body. There may be two wounds, one at the site of entry and one at the site of exit, generally referred to as a "through-and-through."

Closed

Closed wounds have fewer categories, but are just as dangerous as open wounds:

- Hematomas (or blood tumor) – caused by damage to a blood vessel that in turn causes blood to collect under the skin.

  o Hematomas that originate from internal blood vessel pathology are petechiae, purpura, and ecchymosis. The different classifications are based on size.

  o Hematomas that originate from an external source of trauma are contusions, also commonly called bruises.

- Crush injury – caused by a great or extreme amount of force applied over a long period of time.

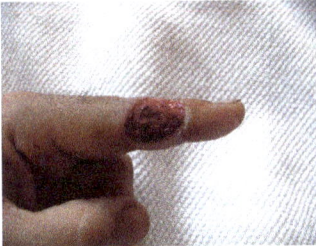
An open wound (an avulsion)

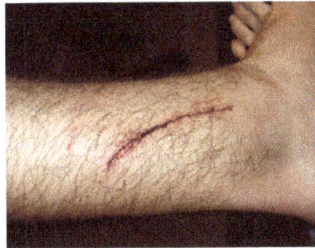
A laceration to the leg

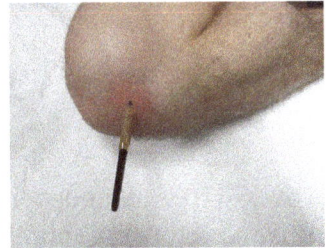
A puncture wound from playing darts.

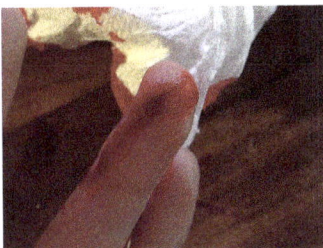
Fresh incisional wound on the fingertip of the left ring finger.

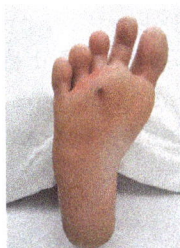
An infected puncture wound to the bottom of the forefoot.

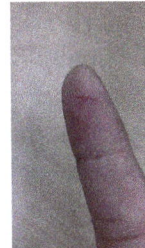
An incision: a small cut in a finger.

Pathophysiology

To heal a wound, the body undertakes a series of actions collectively known as the wound healing process.

Diagnosis

A wound may be recorded for follow-up and observing progress of healing with different techniques which include:

- Photographs, with subsequent area quantification using computer processing

- Wound tracings on acetate sheets

- Kundin wound gauge

Management

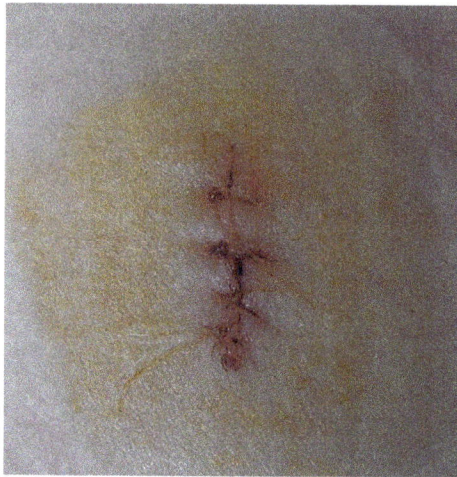

Wound, sewn with four stitches

The overall treatment depends on the type, cause, and depth of the wound, and whether other structures beyond the skin (dermis) are involved. Treatment of recent lacerations involves examining, cleaning, and closing the wound. Minor wounds, like bruises, will heal on their own, with skin discoloration usually disappearing in 1–2 weeks. Abrasions, which are wounds with intact skin (non-penetration through dermis to subcutaneous fat), usually require no active treatment except keeping the area clean, initially with soap and water. Puncture wounds may be prone to infection depending on the depth of penetration. The entry of puncture wound is left open to allow for bacteria or debris to be removed from inside.

Cleaning

Evidence to support the cleaning of wounds before closure is scant. For simple lacerations, cleaning can be accomplished using a number of different solutions, including tap water and sterile saline solution. Infection rates may be lower with the use of tap water in regions where water quality is high. Cleaning of a wound is also known as 'wound toilet'.

Closure

If a person presents to a healthcare center within 6 hours of a laceration they are typically closed immediately after evaluating and cleaning the wound. After this point in time, however, there is a theoretical concern of increased risks of infection if closed immediately. Thus some healthcare providers may delay closure while others may be willing to immediately close up to 24 hours after the injury. Using clean non-sterile gloves is equivalent to using sterile gloves during wound closure.

If closure of a wound is decided upon a number of techniques can be used. These include bandages, a cyanoacrylate glue, staples, and sutures. Absorbable sutures have the benefit over non absorbable sutures of not requiring removal. They are often preferred in children. Buffering the pH of lidocaine makes the injection less painful.

Adhesive glue and sutures have comparable cosmetic outcomes for minor lacerations <5 cm in adults and children. The use of adhesive glue involves considerably less time for the doctor and less pain for the person. The wound opens at a slightly higher rate but there is less redness. The risk for infections (1.1%) is the same for both. Adhesive glue should not be used in areas of high tension or repetitive movements, such as joints or the posterior trunk.

Dressings

In the case of clean surgical wounds, there is no evidence that the use of topical antibiotics reduces infection rates in comparison with non-antibiotic ointment or no ointment at all. Antibiotic ointments can irritate the skin, slow healing, and greatly increase the risk of developing contact dermatitis and antibiotic resistance. Because of this, they should only be used when a person shows signs of infection and not as a preventative.

The effectiveness of dressings and creams containing silver to prevent infection or improve healing is not currently supported by evidence.

Alternative Medicine

There is moderate evidence that honey is more effective than antiseptic followed by gauze for healing wounds infected after surgical operations. There is a lack of quality evidence relating to the use of honey on other types of wounds, such as minor acute wounds, mixed acute and chronic wounds, pressure ulcers, Fournier's gangrene, venous leg ulcers, diabetic foot ulcers and Leishmaniasis.

There is no good evidence that therapeutic touch is useful in healing. More than 400 species of plants are identified as potentially useful for wound healing. Only three randomized controlled trials, however, have been done for the treatment of burns.

An electroactive material developed by NASA has been found beneficial as a wound dressing. It uses electrical activity (generated by body heat and the pressure of cell growth) to facilitate the wound healing process while protecting the wound. The bandage is fabricated from polyvinylidene fluoride, or PVDF, a thermoplastic fluoropolymer that is highly piezoelectric when poled.

Complications

Bacterial infection of wound can impede the healing process and lead to life-threatening complications. Scientists at Sheffield University have used light to rapidly detect the presence of bacteria, by developing a portable kit in which specially designed molecules emit a light signal when bound to bacteria. Current laboratory-based detection of bacteria can take hours or days.

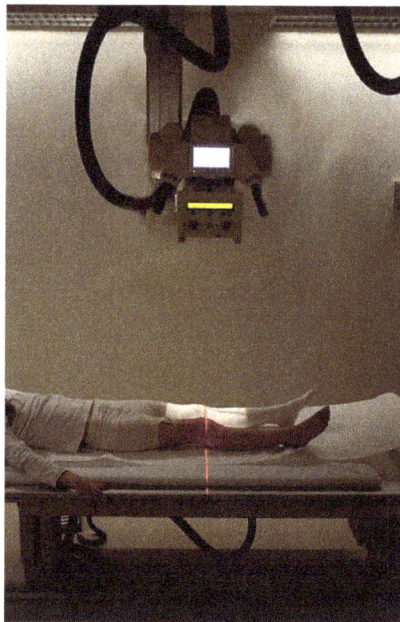

The patient has a deep wound at the knee, and radiography is used to ensure there are no hidden bone fractures.

Workup

Wounds that are not healing should be investigated to find the causes; many microbiological agents may be responsible. The basic workup includes evaluating the wound, its extent and severity. Cultures are usually obtained both from the wound site and blood. X-rays are obtained and a tetanus shot may be administered if there is any doubt about prior vaccination.

Chronic

Non-healing wounds of the diabetic foot are considered one of the most significant complications of diabetes, representing a major worldwide medical, social, and economic burden that greatly affects patient quality of life. Almost 24 million Americans—one in every 12—are diabetic and the disease is causing widespread disability and death at an epidemic pace, according to the Centers for Disease Control and Prevention. Of those with diabetes, 6.5 million are estimated to suffer with chronic or non-healing wounds. Associated with inadequate circulation, poorly functioning veins, and immobility, non-healing wounds occur most frequently in the elderly and in people with diabetes—populations that are sharply rising as the nation ages and chronic diseases increase.

Although diabetes can ravage the body in many ways, non-healing ulcers on the feet and lower legs are common outward manifestations of the disease. Also, diabetics often suffer from nerve damage in their feet and legs, allowing small wounds or irritations to develop without awareness. Given the abnormalities of the microvasculature and other side effects of diabetes, these wounds take a long time to heal and require a specialized treatment approach for proper healing.

As many as 25% of diabetic patients will eventually develop foot ulcers, and recurrence within five years is 70%. If not aggressively treated, these wounds can lead to amputations. It is estimated that every 30 seconds a lower limb is amputated somewhere in the world because of a diabetic wound. Amputation often triggers a downward spiral of declining quality of life, frequently leading to disability and death. In fact, only about one third of diabetic amputees will live more than five years, a survival rate equivalent to that of many cancers.

Many of these lower extremity amputations can be prevented through an interdisciplinary approach to treatment involving a variety of advanced therapies and techniques, such as debridement, hyperbaric oxygen treatment therapy, dressing selection, special shoes, and patient education. When wounds persist, a specialized approach is required for healing.

History

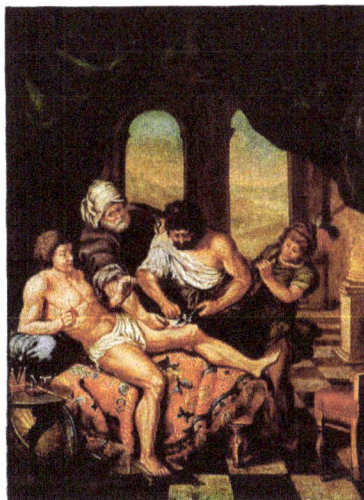

Medieval treatment of wound with lance grittings

From the Classical Period to the Medieval Period, the body and the soul were believed to be intimately connected, based on several theories put forth by the philosopher Plato. Wounds on the body were believed to correlate with wounds to the soul and vice versa; wounds were seen as an outward sign of an inward illness. Thus, a man who was wounded physically in a serious way was said to be hindered not only physically but spiritually as well. If the soul was wounded, that wound may also eventually become physically manifest, revealing the true state of the soul. Wounds were also seen as writing on the "tablet" of the body. Wounds acquired in war, for example, told the story of a soldier in a form which all could see and understand, and the wounds of a martyr told the story of their faith.

Research

In humans and mice it has been shown that estrogen might affect the speed and quality of wound healing

Bruise

A contusion, commonly known as a bruise, is a type of hematoma of tissue in which capillaries and sometimes venules are damaged by trauma, allowing blood to seep, hemorrhage, or extravasate into the surrounding interstitial tissues. Bruises, which do not blanch under pressure, can involve capillaries at the level of skin, subcutaneous tissue, muscle, or bone. Bruises are different from other similar-looking lesions primarily distinguished by their diameter or causation. These lesions include petechia (< 3 mm result from numerous and diverse etiologies such as adverse reactions from medications such as warfarin, straining, asphyxiation, platelet disorders and diseases such as cytomegalovirus), purpura (3 mm to 1 cm, classified as palpable purpura or non-palpable purpura and indicates various pathologic conditions such as thrombocytopenia), and ecchymosis (>1 cm caused blood dissecting through tissue planes and settled in an area remote from the site of trauma or pathology such as periorbital ecchymosis, i.e.,"raccoon eyes" , arising from a basilar skull fracture or from a neuroblastoma).

As a type of hematoma, a bruise is always caused by internal bleeding into the interstitial tissues which does not break through the skin, usually initiated by blunt trauma, which causes damage through physical compression and deceleration forces. Trauma sufficient to cause bruising can occur from a wide variety of situations including accidents, falls, and surgeries. Disease states such as insufficient or malfunctioning platelets, other coagulation deficiencies, or vascular disorders, such as venous blockage associated with severe allergies can lead to the formation of purpura which is different from trauma-related bruising/contusion. If the trauma is sufficient to break the skin and allow blood to escape the interstitial tissues, the injury is not a bruise but instead a different variety of hemorrhage called bleeding. However, such injuries may be accompanied by bruising elsewhere.

Bruises often induce pain, but small bruises are not normally dangerous alone. Sometimes bruises can be serious, leading to other more life-threatening forms of hematoma, such as when associated with serious injuries, including fractures and more severe internal bleeding. The likelihood and severity of bruising depends on many factors, including type and healthiness of affected tissues. Minor bruises may be easily recognized in people with light skin color by characteristic blue or purple appearance (idiomatically described as "black and blue") in the days following the injury.

Cause

The presence of bruises may be seen in patients with platelet or coagulation disorders. Unexplained bruising may be a warning sign of child abuse, domestic abuse, or serious medical problems such as leukemia or meningoccocal infection. Unexplained bruising can also indicate internal bleeding or certain types of cancer. Long-term glucocorticoid therapy can cause easy bruising. Bruising present around the navel (belly button) with severe abdominal pain suggests acute pancreatitis. Connective tissue disorders such as Ehlers-Danlos syndrome may cause relatively easy or spontaneous bruising depending on the severity.

During an autopsy, bruises accompanying abrasions indicate the abrasions occurred while the individual was alive, as opposed to damage incurred post mortem.

Size and Shape

Bruise shapes may correspond directly to the instrument of injury or be modified by additional factors. Bruises often become more prominent as time lapses, resulting in additional size and swelling, and may grow to a large size over the course of the hours after the injury that caused the bruise was inflicted. As stated above, bruising present in a different location than the site of impact is called *ecchymosis* and generally occurs when the tissue at the site of injury is loose, allowing blood to travel under the skin to another location due to gravity or other forces, such as in a black eye.

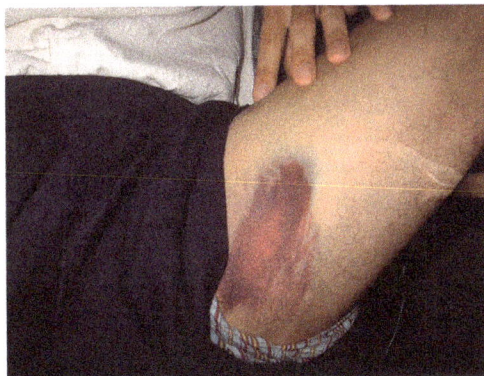

Bruise caused by a handrail, typical of extreme sports

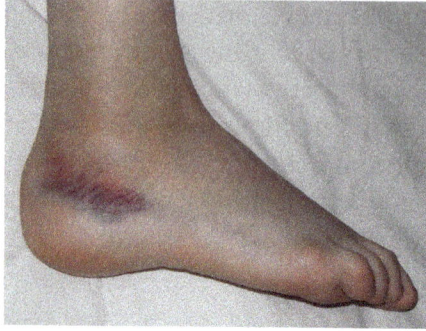

Bruise caused by a sprained ankle

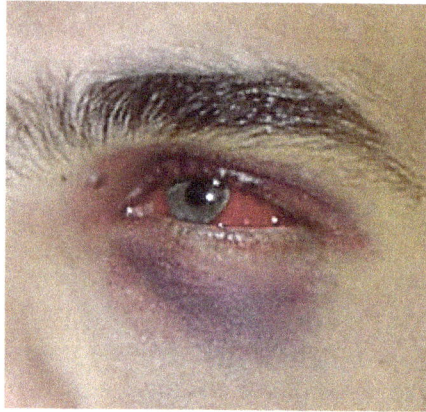

Black eye and subconjunctival hemorrhage after a punch to the face

- Condition and type of tissue: In soft tissues, a larger area is bruised than would be in firmer tissue due to ease of blood to invade tissue.

- Age: elderly skin and other tissues are often thinner and less elastic and thus more prone to bruising.

- Gender: More bruising occurs in females due to increased subcutaneous fat.

- Skin tone: Discoloration caused by bruises is more prominent in lighter complexions.

- Diseases: Coagulation, platelet and blood vessel diseases or deficiencies can increase bruising due to more bleeding.

- Location: More extensive vascularity causes more bleeding. Areas such as the arms, knees, shins and the facial area are especially common bruise sites.

- Forces: Greater striking forces cause greater bruising.

- Genes: Despite having completely normal coagulation factors, natural redheads have been shown to bruise more, although this may just be due to greater visibility on commonly associated lighter complexion.

Severity

Bruises can be scored on a scale from 0-5 to categorize the severity and danger of the injury.

Bruise harm score		
Harm score	**Severity level**	**Notes**
0	Light bruise	No damage
1	Mild bruise	Little damage
2	Moderate bruise	Some damage
3	Serious bruise	Dangerous
4	Extremely serious bruise	Dangerous
5	Critical bruise	Risk of death

The harm score is determined by the extent and severity of the fractures to the organs and tissues causing the bruising, in turn depending on multiple factors. For example, a contracted muscle will bruise more severely, as will tissues crushed against underlying bone. Capillaries vary in strength, stiffness and toughness, which can also vary by age and medical conditions.

An alternate bruise severity ranking system called the Chien Intensity Scale is slowly growing in popularity in some research circles. Although not widely used, the Chien Intensity Scale is used by institutes including the Ryan Mackey Memorial Research Institute and the Sydney Medical Center.

Low levels of damaging forces produce small bruises and generally cause the individual to feel minor pain straight away. Repeated impacts worsen bruises, increasing the harm level. Normally, light bruises heal nearly completely within two weeks, although duration is affected by variation in severity and individual healing processes; generally, more severe or deeper bruises take somewhat longer.

Severe bruising (harm score 2-3) may be dangerous or cause serious complications. Further bleeding and excess fluid may accumulate causing a hard, fluctuating lump or swelling hematoma. This has the potential to cause compartment syndrome as the swelling cuts off blood flow to the tissues. The trauma that induced the bruise may also have caused other severe and potentially fatal harm to internal organs. For example, impacts to the head can cause traumatic brain injury: bleeding, bruising and massive swelling of the brain with the potential to cause concussion, coma and death. Treatment for brain bruising may involve emergency surgery to relieve the pressure on the brain.

Damage that causes bruising can also cause bones to be broken, tendons or muscles to be strained, ligaments to be sprained, or other tissue to be damaged. The symptoms and signs of these injuries may initially appear to be those of simple bruising. Abdominal bruising or severe injuries that cause difficulty in moving a limb or the feeling of liquid under the skin may indicate life-threatening injury and require the attention of a physician.

Mechanism

Increased distress to tissue causes capillaries to break under the skin, allowing blood to escape and build up. As time progresses, blood seeps into the surrounding tissues, causing the bruise to darken and spread. Nerve endings within the affected tissue detect the increased pressure, which, depending on severity and location, may be perceived as pain or pressure or be asymptomatic. The damaged capillary endothelium releases endothelin, a hormone that causes narrowing of the blood vessel to minimize bleeding. As the endothelium is destroyed, the underlying von Willebrand factor is exposed and initiates coagulation, which creates a temporary clot to plug the wound and eventually leads to restoration of normal tissue.

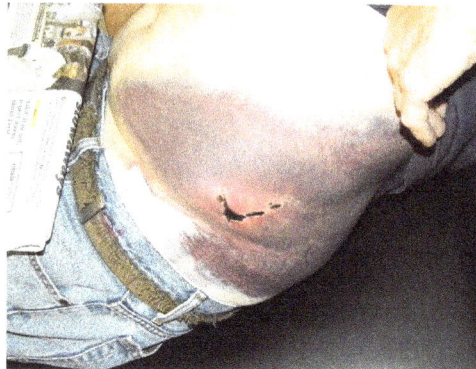

Severe bruising resulting from yard work injury

During this time, larger bruises may change color due to the breakdown of hemoglobin from within escaped red blood cells in the extracellular space. The striking colors of a bruise are caused by the phagocytosis and sequential degradation of hemoglobin to biliverdin to bilirubin to hemosiderin, with hemoglobin itself producing a red-blue color, biliverdin producing a green color, bilirubin producing a yellow color, and hemosiderin producing a golden-brown color. As these products are cleared from the area, the bruise disappears. Often the underlying tissue damage has been repaired long before this process is complete.

Treatment

Treatment for light bruises is minimal and may include RICE (rest, ice, compression, elevation), painkillers (particularly NSAIDs) and, later in recovery, light stretching exercises. Particularly, immediate application of ice while elevating the area may reduce or completely prevent swelling by restricting blood flow to the area and preventing internal bleeding. Rest and preventing re-injury is essential for rapid recovery. Applying a medicated cream containing mucopolysaccharide polysulfuric acid (e.g., Hirudoid) may also speed the healing process. Other topical creams containing skin-fortifying ingredients, including but not limited to retinol or alpha hydroxy acids, such as DerMend, can improve the appearance of bruising faster than if left to heal on its own.

Very gently massaging the area and applying heat may encourage blood flow and relieve pain according to the gate control theory of pain, although causing additional pain may indicate the massage is exacerbating the injury. As for most injuries, these techniques should not be applied until at least three days following the initial damage to ensure all internal bleeding has stopped, because although increasing blood flow will allow more healing factors into the area and encourage drainage, if the injury is still bleeding this will allow more blood to seep out of the wound and cause the bruise to become worse.

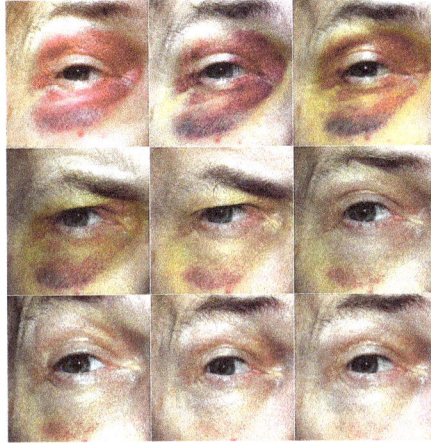

Healing of a black eye over a 9-day period caused by a wisdom tooth extraction

In most cases hematomas spontaneously revert, but in cases of large hematomas or those localized in certain organs (*e.g.*, the brain), the physician may optionally perform a puncture of the hematoma to allow the blood to exit.

History

Folk medicine, including ancient medicine of Egyptians, Greeks, Celts, Turks, Slavs, Mayans, Aztecs and Chinese, has used bruising as a treatment for some health problems. The methods vary widely and include cupping, scraping, and slapping. Fire cupping uses suction which causes bruising in patients. Scraping (Gua Sha) uses a small hand device with a rounded edge to gently scrape the scalp or the skin. Another ancient device that creates mild bruising is a strigil, used by Greeks and Romans in the bath. Archaeologically there is no precedent for scraping tools before Greek archaeological evidence, not Chinese or Egyptian.

Pediatric Trauma

Pediatric trauma refers to a traumatic injury that happens to an infant, child or adolescent. Because of anatomical and physiological differences between children and adults the care and management of this population differs.

Anatomic and Physiologic Differences in Children

There are significant anatomical and physiological differences between children and adults. For example, the internal organs are closer in proximity to each other in children than in adults; this places children at higher risk of traumatic injury.

Children present a unique challenge in trauma care because they are so different from adults - anatomically, developmentally, physiologically and emotionally. A study published in early 2006 in the Journal of Pediatric Surgery concluded that the risk of death for injured children is significantly lower when care is provided in pediatric trauma centers rather than in non-pediatric trauma centers. Yet only about 10% of injured children are treated at pediatric trauma centers. The highest mortality rates occur in children who are treated in rural areas without access trauma centers.

An important part of managing trauma in children is weight estimation. A number of methods to estimate weight exist, including the Broselow tape, Leffler formula, and Theron formula. Of these three methods, the Broselow tape is the most accurate for weight estimation in children ≤25 kg, while the Theron formula performs better with patients weighing >40 kg.

Due to basic geometry, a child's weight to surface area ratio is lower than an adult's, children more readily lose their body heat through radiation and have a higher risk of becoming hypothermic. Smaller body size in children often makes them more prone to poly traumatic injury.

Management

The management of pediatric trauma depends on a knowledge of the physiological, anatomical, and developmental differences in comparison to an adult patient, this requires expertise in this area. In the pre-hospital setting issues may arise with the treatment of pediatric patients due to a lack of knowledge and resources involved in the treatment of these injuries. Despite the fact there is only a slight variation in outcomes in adult trauma centers, definitive care is best reached at a pediatric trauma center.

Pediatric Trauma Score

Several classification systems have been developed that use some combination of subjective and objective data in an effort to quantify the severity of trauma. Examples include the Injury Severity Score and a modified version of the Glasgow Coma Scale. More complex classification systems, such as the Revised Trauma Score, APACHE II, and SAPS II add physiologic data to the equation in an attempt to more precisely define the severity, which can be useful in triaging casualties as well as in determining medical management and predicting prognosis.

Though useful, all of these measures have significant limitations when applied to pediatric patients. For this reason, health care providers often employ classification systems that have been modified or even specifically developed for use in the pediatric population. For example, the Pediatric Glasgow Coma Scale is a modification of the Glasgow Coma Scale that is useful in patients who have not yet developed language skills.

Emphasizing the importance of body weight and airway diameter, the Pediatric Trauma Score (PTS) was developed to specifically reflect the vulnerability of children to traumatic injury. The minimal score is -6 and the maximum score is +12. There is a linear relationship between the decrease in PTS and the mortality risk (i.e. the lower the PTS, the higher the mortality risk). Mortality is estimated at 9% with a PTS > 8, and at 100% with a PTS ≤ 0.

In most cases the severity of a pediatric trauma injury is determined by the pediatric trauma score despite the fact that some research has shown there is no benefit between it and the revised trauma scale.

Epidemiology in the United States

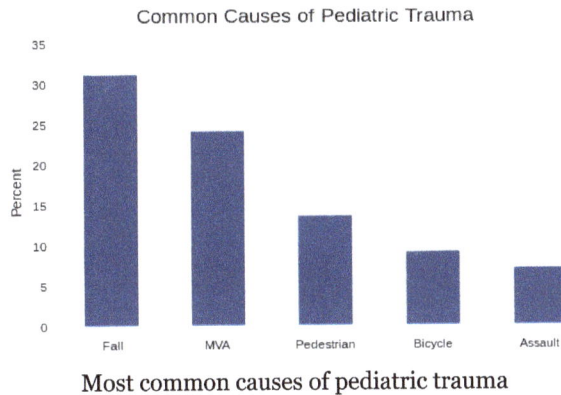

Most common causes of pediatric trauma

Based on the Centers for Disease Control and Prevention's (CDC) WISQARS database for the latest year of data (2010), serious injury kills nearly 10,000 children in America each year.

Pediatric trauma accounted for 59.5% of all mortality for children under 18 in 2004. Injury is the leading cause of death in this age group in the United States—greater than all other causes combined. It is also the leading cause of permanent paralysis for children. In the US approximately 16,000,000 children go to a hospital emergency room due to some kind of injury every year. Male children are more frequently injured than female children by a ratio of two to one. Some injuries, including chemical eye burns, are more common among young children than among their adult counterparts; these are largely due to cleaning supplies and similar chemicals commonly found around the home. Similarly, penetrating injuries in children is because of writing utensils and other common household objects as many are readily available to children in the course of their day.

Blunt Trauma

Blunt trauma, blunt injury, non-penetrating trauma or blunt force trauma refers to physical trauma to a body part, either by impact, injury or physical attack. The latter is usually referred to as blunt force trauma. The term refers to the initial trauma, from which develops more specific types such as contusions, abrasions, lacerations, and/or bone fractures. Blunt trauma is contrasted with penetrating trauma, in which an object such as a bullet enters the body.

Variations

Blunt Abdominal Trauma

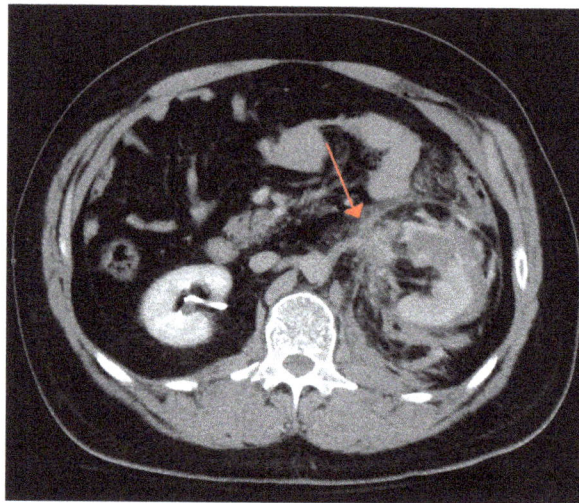

Abdominal CT showing left renal artery injury

Blunt abdominal trauma (BAT) comprises 75% of all blunt trauma and is the most common example of this injury. The majority occurs in motor vehicle accidents, in which rapid deceleration may propel the driver into the steering wheel, dashboard, or seatbelt causing contusions in less serious cases, or rupture of internal organs from briefly increased intraluminal pressure in the more serious, dependent on the force applied. It is important to note that initially there may be little in the way of overt clinical signs to indicate that serious internal abdominal injury has occurred, making assessment more challenging and requiring a high degree of clinical suspicion.

There are two basic physical mechanisms at play with the potential of injury to intra-abdominal organs — compression and deceleration. The former occurs from a direct blow, such as a punch, or compression against a non-yielding object such as a seat belt or steering column. This force may deform a hollow organ thereby increasing its intra-luminal or internal pressure, leading to rupture. Deceleration, on the other hand, causes stretching and shearing at the points at which mobile structures, such as the bowel, are anchored. This can cause tearing of the mesentery of the bowel, and injury to the blood vessels that travel within the mesentery. Classic examples of these mechanisms are a hepatic tear along the ligamentum teres and injuries to the renal arteries.

When blunt abdominal trauma is complicated by 'internal injury', the liver and spleen are most frequently involved, followed by the small intestine.

In rare cases, this injury has been attributed to medical techniques such as the Heimlich Maneuver, attempts at cardiopulmonary resuscitation and manual thrusts to clear an airway. Although these are rare examples, it has been suggested that they are caused by applying unnecessary pressure when administering such techniques. Finally, the occurrence of splenic rupture with mild blunt abdominal trama in those convalescing from infectious mononucleosis is well reported.

Diagnosis

In all but the most obviously trivial injuries, the first concern is to exclude anything that might be quickly or immediately life-threatening. This is resolved by ascertaining that the subject's airway is open and competent, that breathing is unlabored, and that circulation — i.e. pulses that can be felt, is present. This is sometimes described as the "A, B, C's" — Airway, Breathing, and Circulation – and is the first step in any resuscitation or triage. Then, the history of the accident or injury is amplified with any medical, dietary (timing of last oral intake) and past history, from whatever sources such as family, friends, previous treating physicians that might be available. This method is sometimes given the mnemonic "SAMPLE". The amount of time spent on diagnosis should be minimized and expedited by a combination of clinical assessment and appropriate use of technology, such as diagnostic peritoneal lavage (DPL), or bedside ultrasound examination (FAST) before proceeding to laparotomy if required. If time and the patient's stability permits, CT examination may be carried out if available. Its advantages include superior definition of the injury, leading to grading of the injury and sometimes the confidence to avoid or postpone surgery. Its disadvantages include the time taken to acquire images — although this gets shorter with each generation of scanners — and the removal of the patient from the immediate view of the emergency or surgical staff.

Recently, criteria have been defined that might allow patients with blunt abdominal trauma to be discharged safely without further evaluation. The characteristics of such patients would include:

- absence of intoxication

- no evidence of lowered blood pressure or raised pulse rate

- no abdominal pain or tenderness

- no blood in the urine.

To be considered low risk, patients would need to meet all low-risk criteria.

Blunt Abdominal Trauma in Sports

In the United States, the majority of contact-collision injuries, usually blunt trauma, should have been witnessed in high school or collegiate games where the athletic training staff are trained to keep their eyes on the play. This may allow some departure from Advanced Trauma Life Support guidelines in the initial assessment, although the principles always apply. The major priority then becomes separating contusions and musculo-tendinous injuries from injuries to solid organs and the gut and recognizing potential or developing blood loss, and reacting accordingly. Blunt injuries to the kidney from helmets, shoulder pads, and knees are also described in American football, association football, martial arts, and all-terrain vehicle accidents.

Treatment

In every case where the presumption of internal injury has been sufficient to trigger the diagnostic steps outlined above, intravenous access will be established and crystalloid solutions and/or blood will be administered at rates sufficient to maintain the circulation. Thereafter, further treatment will depend on the grade of organ damage estimated by the prior investigations and will vary from close observation with the ability to intervene quickly, or surgery, open or laparoscopic. In the case of blunt adbominal trauma, there is no shown benefit from surgery unless active bleeding is present.

Penetrating Trauma

Penetrating trauma is an injury that occurs when an object pierces the skin and enters a tissue of the body, creating an open wound. In blunt, or non-penetrating trauma, there may be an impact, but the skin is not necessarily broken. The penetrating object may remain in the tissues, come back out the way it entered, or pass through the tissues and exit from another area. An injury in which an object enters the body or a structure and passes all the way through is called a perforating injury, while *penetrating trauma* implies that the object does not pass through. Perforating trauma is associated with an entrance wound and an often larger exit wound.

Penetrating trauma can be caused by a foreign object or by fragments of a broken bone. Usually occurring in violent crime or armed combat, penetrating injuries are commonly caused by gunshots and stabbings.

Penetrating trauma can be serious because it can damage internal organs and presents a risk of shock and infection. The severity of the injury varies widely depending on the body parts involved, the characteristics of the penetrating object, and the amount of energy transmitted to the tissues. Assessment may involve X-rays or CT scans, and treatment may involve surgery, for example to repair damaged structures or to remove foreign objects.

Puncture and penetration are similar however a puncture is different from a penetration wound in that there is no exit wound in cases of puncture. This type of trauma can be seen for example in a stabbing, or a gunshot wound in which a low velocity pistol bullet was used.

Mechanism

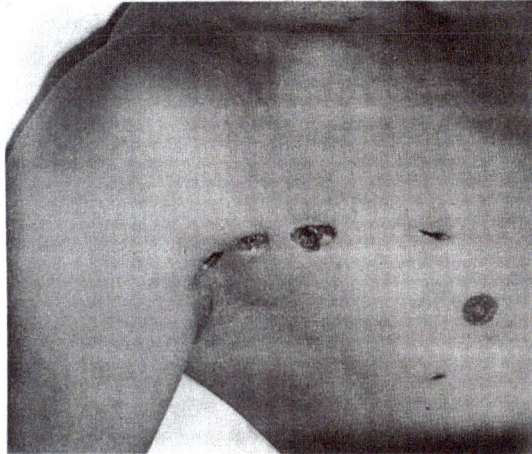

FIGURE 1.—Superficial bullet wounds of chest wall not involving bony structures.

A gunshot wound

As a missile passes through tissue, it decelerates, dissipating and transferring kinetic energy to the tissues; this is what causes the injury. The velocity of the projectile is a more important factor than its mass in determining how much damage is done; kinetic energy increases with the square of the velocity. In addition to injury caused directly by the object that enters the body, penetrating injuries may be associated with secondary injuries, due for example to a blast injury. High-velocity objects are usually projectiles such as bullets from high-powered rifles, such as assault rifles or sniper rifles. Bullets classed as medium-velocity projectiles include those from handguns, shotguns, and submachine guns. Low-velocity items, such as knives and swords, are usually propelled by a person's hand, and usually do damage only to the area that is directly contacted by the object. The space left by tissue that is destroyed by the penetrating object as it passes through forms a cavity; this is called permanent cavitation. In addition to causing damage to the tissues they contact, medium- and high-velocity projectiles cause a secondary cavitation injury: as the object enters the body, it creates a pressure wave which forces tissue out of the way, creating a "temporary cavity" that can be much larger than the object itself. The tissues soon move back into place, eliminating the cavity, but the cavitation frequently does considerable damage first. Temporary cavitation can be especially damaging when it affects delicate tissues such as the brain, as occurs in penetrating head trauma.

The characteristics of the tissue injured also help determine the severity of the injury; for example, the denser the tissue, the greater the amount of energy transmitted to it. The path of a projectile can be estimated by imagining a line from the entrance wound to the exit wound, but the actual trajectory may vary due to ricochet or differences in tissue density. In a cut, the discolouration and the swelling of the skin from a blow happens because of the ruptured blood vessels and escape of blood and fluid and other injury that interrupts the circulation.

Head

While penetrating head trauma accounts for only a small percentage of all traumatic brain injuries, it is associated with a high mortality rate, and only a third of people with penetrating head trauma survive long enough to arrive at a hospital. Injuries from firearms are the leading cause of TBI-related deaths. Penetrating head trauma can cause cerebral contusions and lacerations, intracranial hematomas, pseudoaneurysms, and arteriovenous fistulas. The prognosis for penetrating head injuries varies widely.

Penetrating facial trauma can pose a risk to the airway and breathing; airway obstruction can occur later due to swelling or bleeding. Penetrating eye trauma can cause the globe of the eye to rupture or vitreous humor to leak from it, and presents a serious threat to eyesight.

Chest

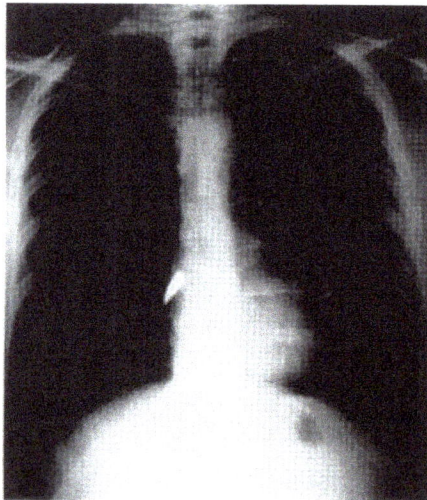

X-ray showing a bullet (white spot) in the heart

Most penetrating injuries are chest wounds and have a mortality rate (death rate) of under 10%. Penetrating chest trauma can injure vital organs such as the heart and lungs and can interfere with breathing and circulation. Lung injuries that can be caused by penetrating trauma include pulmonary laceration (a cut or tear) pulmonary contusion (a bruise), hemothorax (an accumulation of blood in the chest cavity outside of the lung), pneumothorax (an accumulation of air in the chest cavity) and hemopneumothorax (accumulation of both blood and air). Sucking chest wounds and tension pneumothorax may result.

Penetrating trauma can also cause injuries to the heart and circulatory system. When the heart is punctured, it may bleed profusely into the chest cavity if the membrane around it (the pericardium) is significantly torn, or it may cause pericardial tamponade if the pericardium is not disrupted. In pericardial tamponade, blood escapes from the heart but is trapped within the pericardium, so pressure builds up between the pericardium and the heart, compressing the latter and interfering with its pumping. Fractures of the ribs commonly produce penetrating chest trauma when sharp bone ends pierce tissues.

Abdomen

Penetrating abdominal trauma (PAT) typically arises from stabbings, ballistic injuries (shootings), or industrial accidents. PAT can be life-threatening because abdominal organs, especially those in the retroperitoneal space, can bleed profusely, and the space can hold a large volume of blood. If the pancreas is injured, it may be further injured by its own secretions, in a process called *autodigestion*. Injuries of the liver, common because of the size and location of the organ, present a serious risk for shock because the liver tissue is delicate and has a large blood supply and capacity. The intestines, taking a large part of the lower abdomen, are also at risk of perforation.

People with penetrating abdominal trauma may have signs of hypovolemic shock (insufficient blood in the circulatory system) and peritonitis (an inflammation of the peritoneum, the membrane that lines the abdominal cavity). Penetration may abolish or diminish bowel sounds due to bleeding, infection, and irritation, and injuries to arteries may cause bruits (a distinctive sound similar to heart murmurs) to be audible. Percussion of the abdomen may reveal hyperresonance (indicating air in the abdominal cavity) or dullness (indicating a buildup of blood). The abdomen may be distended or tender, signs which indicate an urgent need for surgery.

The standard management of penetrating abdominal trauma was for many years mandatory laparotomy. A greater understanding of mechanisms of injury, outcomes from surgery, improved imaging and interventional radiology has led to more conservative operative strategies being adopted.

Assessment and Treatment

Assessment can be difficult because much of the damage is often internal and not visible. The patient is thoroughly examined. X-ray and CT scanning may be used to identify the type and location of potentially lethal injuries. Sometimes before an X-ray is performed on a person with penetrating trauma from a projectile, a paper clip is taped over entry and exit wounds to show their location on the film. The patient is given intravenous fluids to replace lost blood. Surgery may be required; impaled objects are secured into place so that they do not move and cause further injury, and they are removed in an operating room. Foreign bodies such as bullets may be removed, but they may also be left in place if the surgery necessary to get them out would cause more damage than would leaving them. Wounds are debrided to remove tissue that cannot survive and other material that presents risk for infection.

History

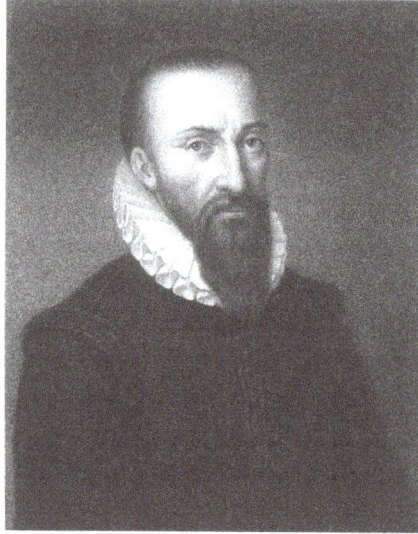

Ambroise Paré

Before the 17th century, medical practitioners poured hot oil into wounds in order to cauterize damaged blood vessels, but the French surgeon Ambroise Paré challenged the use of this method in 1545. Paré was the first to propose controlling bleeding using ligature.

During the American Civil War, chloroform was used during surgery to reduce pain and allow more time for operations. Due in part to the lack of sterile technique in hospitals, infection was the leading cause of death for wounded soldiers.

In World War I, doctors began replacing patients' lost fluid with salt solutions. With World War II came the idea of blood banking, having quantities of donated blood available to replace lost fluids. The use of antibiotics also came into practice in World War II.

Cardiac Tamponade

Cardiac tamponade, also known as pericardial tamponade, is when fluid in the pericardium (the sac around the heart) builds up and results in compression of the heart. Onset may be rapid or more gradual. Symptoms typically include those of cardiogenic shock including shortness of breath, weakness, lightheadedness, and cough. Other symptoms may relate to the underlying cause.

Common causes include cancer, kidney failure, chest trauma, and pericarditis. Other causes include connective tissue diseases, hypothyroidism, aortic rupture, and following cardiac surgery. In Africa, tuberculosis is a relatively common cause.

Diagnosis may be suspected based on low blood pressure, jugular venous distension, pericardial rub, or quiet heart sounds. The diagnosis may be further supported by specific electrocardiogram (ECG) changes, chest X-ray, or an ultrasound of the heart. If fluid increases slowly the pericardial sac can expand to contain more than 2 liters; however, if the increase is rapid as little as 200 mL can result in tamponade.

When tamponade results in symptoms, drainage is necessary. This can be done by pericardiocentesis, surgery to create a pericardial window, or a pericardiectomy. Drainage may also be necessary to rule out infection or cancer. Other treatments may include the use of dobutamine or in those with low blood volume, intravenous fluids. Those with few symptoms and no worrisome features can often be closely followed. The frequency of tamponade is unclear. One estimate from the United States places it at 2 per 10,000 per year.

Signs and Symptoms

Onset may be rapid or more gradual. Symptoms typically include those of cardiogenic shock including shortness of breath, weakness, lightheadedness, and cough. Other symptoms may relate to the underlying cause.

Causes

Cardiac tamponade is caused by a large or uncontrolled pericardial effusion, i.e. the buildup of fluid inside the pericardium. This commonly occurs as a result of chest trauma (both blunt and penetrating), but can also be caused by myocardial rupture, cancer, uremia, pericarditis, or cardiac surgery, and rarely occurs during retrograde aortic dissection, or while the person is taking anticoagulant therapy. The effusion can occur rapidly (as in the case of trauma or myocardial rupture), or over a more gradual period of time (as in cancer). The fluid involved is often blood, but pus is also found in some circumstances.

Causes of increased pericardial effusion include hypothyroidism, physical trauma (either penetrating trauma involving the pericardium or blunt chest trauma), pericarditis (inflammation of the pericardium), iatrogenic trauma (during an invasive procedure), and myocardial rupture.

Surgery

One of the most common settings for cardiac tamponade is in the first 24 to 48 hours after heart surgery. After heart surgery, chest tubes are placed to drain blood. These chest tubes, however, are prone to clot formation. When a chest tube becomes occluded or clogged, the blood that should be drained can accumulate around the heart, leading to tamponade.

Pathophysiology

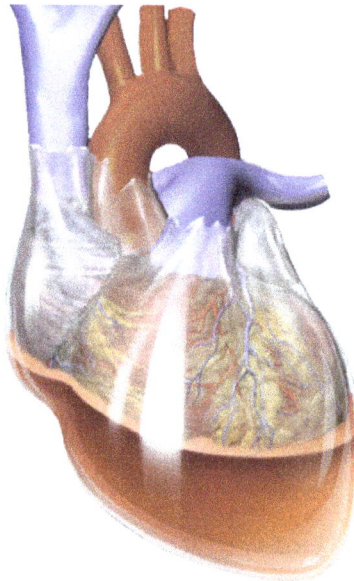

Hemopericardium, wherein the pericardium becomes filled with blood, is one cause of cardiac tamponade.

The outer layer of the heart is made of fibrous tissue which does not easily stretch, so once fluid begins to enter the pericardial space, pressure starts to increase.

If fluid continues to accumulate, each successive diastolic period leads to less blood entering the ventricles. Eventually, increasing pressure on the heart forces the septum to bend in towards the left ventricle, leading to a decrease in stroke volume. This causes the development of obstructive shock, which if left untreated may lead to cardiac arrest (often presenting as pulseless electrical activity).

Diagnosis

Initial diagnosis can be challenging, as there are a number of differential diagnoses, including tension pneumothorax, and acute heart failure. In a trauma patient presenting with PEA (pulseless electrical activity) in the absence of hypovolemia and tension pneumothorax, the most likely diagnosis is cardiac tamponade.

Signs of classical cardiac tamponade include three signs, known as Beck's triad. Low blood pressure occurs because of decreased stroke volume, jugular-venous distension due to impaired venous return to the heart, and muffled heart sounds due to fluid buildup inside the pericardium.

Other signs of tamponade include pulsus paradoxus (a drop of at least 10 mmHg in arterial blood pressure with inspiration), and ST segment changes on the electrocardiogram, which may also show low voltage QRS complexes, as well as general signs and symptoms of shock (such as fast heart rate, shortness of breath and decreasing level of consciousness). However, some of these signs may not be present in certain cases. A fast heart rate, although expected, may be absent in people with uremia and hypothyroidism.

In addition to the diagnostic complications afforded by the wide-ranging differential diagnosis for chest pain, diagnosis can be additionally complicated by the fact that patients will often be weak or faint at presentation. For instance, a fast rate of breathing and difficulty breathing on exertion that progresses to air hunger at rest can be a key diagnostic symptom, but it may not be possible to obtain such information from patients who are unconscious or who have convulsions at presentation.

Tamponade can often be diagnosed radiographically. Echocardiography, which is the diagnostic test of choice, often demonstrates an enlarged pericardium or collapsed ventricles. A large cardiac tamponade will show as an enlarged globular-shaped heart on chest x-ray. During inspiration, the negative pressure in the thoracic cavity will cause increased pressure into the right ventricle. This increased pressure in the right ventricle will cause the interventricular septum to bulge towards the left ventricle, leading to decreased filling of the left ventricle. At the same time, right ventricle volume is markedly diminished and sometimes it can collapse.

Treatment

Pre-hospital Care

Initial treatment given will usually be supportive in nature, for example administration of oxygen, and monitoring. There is little care that can be provided pre-hospital other than general treatment for shock. Some teams have performed an emergency thoracotomy to release clotting in the pericardium caused by a penetrating chest injury.

Prompt diagnosis and treatment is the key to survival with tamponade. Some pre-hospital providers will have facilities to provide pericardiocentesis, which can be life-saving. If the patient has already suffered a cardiac arrest, pericardiocentesis alone cannot ensure survival, and so rapid evacuation to a hospital is usually the more appropriate course of action.

Hospital Management

Initial management in hospital is by pericardiocentesis. This involves the insertion of a needle through the skin and into the pericardium and aspirating fluid under ultrasound guidance preferably. This can be done laterally through the intercostal spaces, usually the fifth, or as a subxiphoid approach. A left parasternal approach begins 3 to 5 cm left of the sternum to avoid the left internal mammary artery, in the 5th intercostal space. Often, a cannula is left in place during resuscitation following initial drainage so that the procedure can be performed again if the need arises. If facilities are available, an emergency pericardial window may be performed instead, during which the pericardium is cut open to allow fluid to drain. Following stabilization of the patient, surgery is provided to seal the source of the bleed and mend the pericardium.

In people following heart surgery the nurses monitor the amount of chest tube drainage. If the drainage volume drops off, and the blood pressure goes down, this can suggest tamponade due to chest tube clogging. In that case, the patient is taken back to the operating room for an emergency reoperation.

If aggressive treatment is offered immediately and no complications arise (shock, AMI or arrhythmia, heart failure, aneurysm, carditis, embolism, or rupture), or they are dealt with quickly and fully contained, then adequate survival is still a distinct possibility.

Epidemiology

The frequency of tamponade is unclear. One estimate from the United States places it at 2 per 10,000 per year. It is estimated to occur in 2% of those with stab or gunshot wounds to the chest.

Stroke

A stroke is when poor blood flow to the brain results in cell death. There are two main types of stroke: ischemic, due to lack of blood flow, and hemorrhagic, due to bleeding. They result in part of the brain not functioning properly. Signs and symptoms of a stroke may include an inability to move or feel on one side of the body, problems understanding or speaking, feeling like the world is spinning, or loss of vision to one side. Signs and symptoms often appear soon after the stroke has occurred. If symptoms last less than one or two hours it is known as a transient ischemic attack (TIA) or ministroke. A hemorrhagic stroke may also be associated with a severe headache. The symptoms of a stroke can be permanent. Long-term complications may include pneumonia or loss of bladder control.

The main risk factor for stroke is high blood pressure. Other risk factors include tobacco smoking, obesity, high blood cholesterol, diabetes mellitus, previous TIA, and atrial fibrillation. An ischemic stroke is typically caused by blockage of a blood vessel, though there are also less common causes. A hemorrhagic stroke is caused by either bleeding directly into the brain or into the space between the brain's membranes. Bleeding may occur due to a ruptured brain aneurysm. Diagnosis is typically with medical imaging such as a CT scan or magnetic resonance imaging (MRI) scan along with a physical exam. Other tests such as an electrocardiogram (ECG) and blood tests are done to determine risk factors and rule out other possible causes. Low blood sugar may cause similar symptoms.

Prevention includes decreasing risk factors, as well as possibly aspirin, statins, surgery to open up the arteries to the brain in those with problematic narrowing, and warfarin in those with atrial fibrillation. A stroke or TIA often requires emergency care. An ischemic stroke, if detected within three to four and half hours, may be treatable with a medication that can break down the clot. Aspirin should be used. Some hemorrhagic strokes benefit from surgery. Treatment to try to recover lost function is called stroke rehabilitation and ideally takes place in a stroke unit; however, these are not available in much of the world.

In 2013 approximately 6.9 million people had an ischemic stroke and 3.4 million people had a hemorrhagic stroke. In 2015 there were about 42.4 million people who had previously had a stroke and were still alive. Between 1990 and 2010 the number of strokes which occurred each year decreased by approximately 10% in the developed world and increased by 10% in the developing world. In 2015, stroke was the second most frequent cause of death after coronary artery disease, accounting for 6.3 million deaths (11% of the total). About 3.0 million deaths resulted from ischemic stroke while 3.3 million deaths resulted from hemorrhagic stroke. About half of people who have had a stroke live less than one year. Overall, two thirds of strokes occurred in those over 65 years old.

Classification

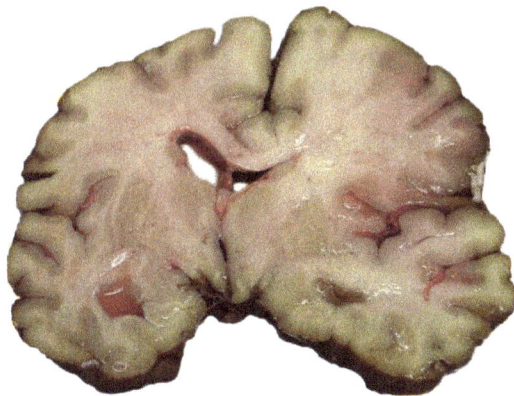

A slice of brain from the autopsy of a person who had an acute middle cerebral artery (MCA) stroke

Strokes can be classified into two major categories: ischemic and hemorrhagic. Ischemic strokes are caused by interruption of the blood supply to the brain, while hemorrhagic strokes result from the rupture of a blood vessel or an abnormal vascular structure. About 87% of strokes are ischemic, the rest being hemorrhagic. Bleeding can develop inside areas of ischemia, a condition known as "hemorrhagic transformation." It is unknown how many hemorrhagic strokes actually start as ischemic strokes.

Definition

In the 1970s the World Health Organization defined stroke as a "neurological deficit of cerebrovascular cause that persists beyond 24 hours or is interrupted by death within 24 hours", although the word "stroke" is centuries old. This definition was supposed to reflect the reversibility of tissue damage and was devised for the purpose, with the time frame of 24 hours being chosen arbitrarily. The 24-hour limit divides stroke from transient ischemic attack, which is a related syndrome of stroke symptoms that resolve completely within 24 hours. With the availability of treatments which can reduce stroke severity when given early, many now prefer alternative terminology, such as brain attack and acute ischemic cerebrovascular syndrome (modeled after heart attack and acute coronary syndrome, respectively), to reflect the urgency of stroke symptoms and the need to act swiftly.

Ischemic

In an ischemic stroke, blood supply to part of the brain is decreased, leading to dysfunction of the brain tissue in that area. There are four reasons why this might happen:

1. Thrombosis (obstruction of a blood vessel by a blood clot forming locally)

2. Embolism (obstruction due to an embolus from elsewhere in the body),

3. Systemic hypoperfusion (general decrease in blood supply, e.g., in shock)

4. cerebral venous sinus thrombosis.

Stroke without an obvious explanation is termed "cryptogenic" (of unknown origin); this constitutes 30-40% of all ischemic strokes.

There are various classification systems for acute ischemic stroke. The Oxford Community Stroke Project classification (OCSP, also known as the Bamford or Oxford classification) relies primarily on the initial symptoms; based on the extent of the symptoms, the stroke episode is classified as total anterior circulation infarct (TACI), partial anterior circulation infarct (PACI), lacunar infarct (LACI) or posterior circulation infarct (POCI). These four entities predict the extent of the stroke, the area of the brain that is affected, the underlying cause, and the prognosis. The TOAST (Trial of Org 10172 in Acute Stroke Treatment) classification is based on clinical symptoms as well as results of further investigations; on this basis, a stroke is classified as being due to (1) thrombosis or embolism due to atherosclerosis of a large artery, (2) an embolism originating in the heart, (3) complete blockage of a small blood vessel, (4) other determined cause, (5) undetermined cause (two possible causes, no cause identified, or incomplete investigation). Users of stimulants, such as cocaine and methamphetamine are at a high risk for ischemic strokes.

Hemorrhagic

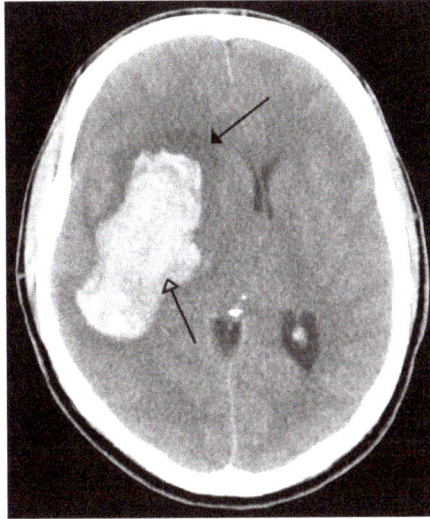

CT scan of an intraparenchymal bleed (bottom arrow) with surrounding edema (top arrow)

There are two main types of hemorrhagic stroke:

- Cerebral hemorrhage (also known as intracerebral hemorrhage), which is basically bleeding within the brain itself (when an artery in the brain bursts, flooding the surrounding tissue with blood), due to either intraparenchymal hemorrhage (bleeding within the brain tissue) or intraventricular hemorrhage (bleeding within the brain's ventricular system).

- Subarachnoid hemorrhage, which is basically bleeding that occurs outside of the brain tissue but still within the skull, and precisely between the arachnoid mater and pia mater (the delicate *innermost* layer of the three layers of the meninges that surround the brain).

The above two main types of hemorrhagic stroke are also two different forms of intracranial hemorrhage, which is the accumulation of blood anywhere within the cranial vault; but the other forms of intracranial hemorrhage, such as epidural hematoma (bleeding between the skull and the dura mater, which is the thick *outermost* layer of the meninges that surround the brain) and subdural hematoma (bleeding in the subdural space), are not considered "hemorrhagic strokes".

Hemorrhagic strokes may occur on the background of alterations to the blood vessels in the brain, such as cerebral amyloid angiopathy, cerebral arteriovenous malformation and an intracranial aneurysm, which can cause intraparenchymal or subarachnoid hemorrhage.

In addition to neurological impairment, hemorrhagic strokes usually cause specific symptoms (for instance, subarachnoid hemorrhage classically causes a severe headache known as a thunderclap headache) or reveal evidence of a previous head injury.

Signs and Symptoms

Stroke symptoms typically start suddenly, over seconds to minutes, and in most cases do not progress further. The symptoms depend on the area of the brain affected. The more extensive the area of the brain affected, the more functions that are likely to be lost. Some forms of stroke can cause additional symptoms. For example, in intracranial hemorrhage, the affected area may compress other structures. Most forms of stroke are not associated with a headache, apart from subarachnoid hemorrhage and cerebral venous thrombosis and occasionally intracerebral hemorrhage.

Early Recognition

Various systems have been proposed to increase recognition of stroke. Different findings are able to predict the presence or absence of stroke to different degrees. Sudden-onset face weakness, arm drift (i.e., if a person, when asked to raise both arms, involuntarily lets one arm drift downward) and abnormal speech are the findings most likely to lead to the correct identification of a case of stroke increasing the likelihood by 5.5 when at least one of these is present). Similarly, when all three of these are absent, the likelihood of stroke is significantly decreased (– likelihood ratio of 0.39). While these findings are not perfect for diagnosing stroke, the fact that they can be evaluated relatively rapidly and easily make them very valuable in the acute setting.

A mnemonic to remember the warning signs of stroke is FAST (facial droop, arm weakness, speech difficulty, and time to call emergency services), as advocated by the Department of Health (United Kingdom) and the Stroke Association, the American Stroke Association, the National Stroke Association (US), the Los Angeles Prehospital Stroke Screen (LAPSS) and the Cincinnati Prehospital Stroke Scale (CPSS). Use of these scales is recommended by professional guidelines.

For people referred to the emergency room, early recognition of stroke is deemed important as this can expedite diagnostic tests and treatments. A scoring system called ROSIER (recognition of stroke in the emergency room) is recommended for this purpose; it is based on features from the medical history and physical examination.

Subtypes

If the area of the brain affected contains one of the three prominent central nervous system pathways—the spinothalamic tract, corticospinal tract, and dorsal column (medial lemniscus), symptoms may include:

- hemiplegia and muscle weakness of the face

- numbness

- reduction in sensory or vibratory sensation

- initial flaccidity (reduced muscle tone), replaced by spasticity (increased muscle tone), excessive reflexes, and obligatory synergies.

In most cases, the symptoms affect only one side of the body (unilateral). Depending on the part of the brain affected, the defect in the brain is *usually* on the opposite side of the body. However, since these pathways also travel in the spinal cord and any lesion there can also produce these symptoms, the presence of any one of these symptoms does not necessarily indicate a stroke.In addition to the above CNS pathways, the *brainstem* gives rise to most of the twelve cranial nerves. A brainstem stroke affecting the brainstem and brain, therefore, can produce symptoms relating to deficits in these cranial nerves:

- altered smell, taste, hearing, or vision (total or partial)

- drooping of eyelid (ptosis) and weakness of ocular muscles

- decreased reflexes: gag, swallow, pupil reactivity to light

- decreased sensation and muscle weakness of the face

- balance problems and nystagmus

- altered breathing and heart rate

- weakness in sternocleidomastoid muscle with inability to turn head to one side

- weakness in tongue (inability to stick out the tongue and/or move it from side to side)

If the *cerebral cortex* is involved, the CNS pathways can again be affected, but also can produce the following symptoms:

- aphasia (difficulty with verbal expression, auditory comprehension, reading and/or writing; Broca's or Wernicke's area typically involved)

- dysarthria (motor speech disorder resulting from neurological injury)

- apraxia (altered voluntary movements)

- visual field defect

- memory deficits (involvement of temporal lobe)

- hemineglect (involvement of parietal lobe)

- disorganized thinking, confusion, hypersexual gestures (with involvement of frontal lobe)

- lack of insight of his or her, usually stroke-related, disability

If the *cerebellum* is involved, ataxia might be present and this includes:

- altered walking gait

- altered movement coordination

- vertigo and or disequilibrium

Associated Symptoms

Loss of consciousness, headache, and vomiting usually occur more often in hemorrhagic stroke than in thrombosis because of the increased intracranial pressure from the leaking blood compressing the brain.

If symptoms are maximal at onset, the cause is more likely to be a subarachnoid hemorrhage or an embolic stroke.

Causes

Thrombotic Stroke

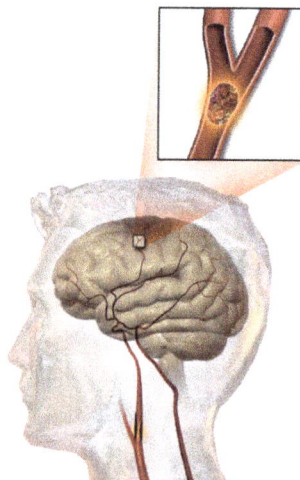

Illustration of an embolic stroke, showing a blockage lodged in a blood vessel.

In thrombotic stroke, a thrombus (blood clot) usually forms around atherosclerotic plaques. Since blockage of the artery is gradual, onset of symptomatic thrombotic strokes is slower than that of a hemorrhagic stroke. A thrombus itself (even if it does not completely block the blood vessel) can lead to an embolic stroke if the thrombus breaks off and travels in the bloodstream, at which point it is called an embolus. Two types of thrombosis can cause stroke:

- *Large vessel disease* involves the common and internal carotid arteries, the vertebral artery, and the Circle of Willis. Diseases that may form thrombi in the large vessels include (in descending incidence): atherosclerosis, vasoconstriction (tightening of the artery), aortic, carotid or vertebral artery dissection, various inflammatory diseases of the blood vessel wall (Takayasu arteritis, giant cell arteritis, vasculitis), noninflammatory vasculopathy, Moyamoya disease and fibromuscular dysplasia.

- *Small vessel disease* involves the smaller arteries inside the brain: branches of the circle of Willis, middle cerebral artery, stem, and arteries arising from the distal vertebral and basilar artery. Diseases that may form thrombi in the small vessels include (in descending incidence): lipohyalinosis (build-up of fatty hyaline matter in the blood vessel as a result of high blood pressure and aging) and fibrinoid degeneration (a stroke involving these vessels are known as a lacunar stroke) and microatheroma (small atherosclerotic plaques).

Sickle-cell anemia, which can cause blood cells to clump up and block blood vessels, can also lead to stroke. A stroke is the second leading cause of death in people under 20 with sickle-cell anemia. Air pollution may also increase stroke risk.

Embolic Stroke

An embolic stroke refers to an arterial embolism (a blockage of an artery) by an embolus, a traveling particle or debris in the arterial bloodstream originating from elsewhere. An embolus is most frequently a thrombus, but it can also be a number of other substances including fat (e.g., from bone marrow in a broken bone), air, cancer cells or clumps of bacteria (usually from infectious endocarditis).

Because an embolus arises from elsewhere, local therapy solves the problem only temporarily. Thus, the source of the embolus must be identified. Because the embolic blockage is sudden in onset, symptoms usually are maximal at the start. Also, symptoms may be transient as the embolus is partially resorbed and moves to a different location or dissipates altogether.

Emboli most commonly arise from the heart (especially in atrial fibrillation) but may originate from elsewhere in the arterial tree. In paradoxical embolism, a deep vein thrombosis embolizes through an atrial or ventricular septal defect in the heart into the brain.

Causes of stroke related to the heart can be distinguished between high and low-risk:

- High risk: atrial fibrillation and paroxysmal atrial fibrillation, rheumatic disease of the mitral or aortic valve disease, artificial heart valves, known cardiac thrombus of the atrium or ventricle, sick sinus syndrome, sustained atrial flutter, recent myocardial infarction, chronic myocardial infarction together with ejection fraction <28 percent, symptomatic congestive heart failure with ejection fraction <30 percent, dilated cardiomyopathy, Libman-Sacks endocarditis, Marantic endocarditis, infective endocarditis, papillary fibroelastoma, left atrial myxoma and coronary artery bypass graft (CABG) surgery.

- Low risk/potential: calcification of the annulus (ring) of the mitral valve, patent foramen ovale (PFO), atrial septal aneurysm, atrial septal aneurysm *with* patent foramen ovale, left ventricular aneurysm without thrombus, isolated left atrial "smoke" on echocardiography (no mitral stenosis or atrial fibrillation), complex atheroma in the ascending aorta or proximal arch.

Among those who have a complete blockage of one of the carotid arteries, the risk of stroke on that side is about one percent per year.

Cerebral Hypoperfusion

Cerebral hypoperfusion is the reduction of blood flow to all parts of the brain. The reduction could be to a particular part of the brain depending on the cause. It is most commonly due to heart failure from cardiac arrest or arrhythmias, or from reduced cardiac output as a result of myocardial infarction, pulmonary embolism, pericardial effusion, or bleeding. Hypoxemia (low blood oxygen content) may precipitate the hypoperfusion. Because the reduction in blood flow is global, all parts of the brain may be affected, especially vulnerable "watershed" areas - border zone regions supplied by the major cerebral arteries. A watershed stroke refers to the condition when the blood supply to these areas is compromised. Blood flow to these areas does not necessarily stop, but instead it may lessen to the point where brain damage can occur.

Venous Thrombosis

Cerebral venous sinus thrombosis leads to stroke due to locally increased venous pressure, which exceeds the pressure generated by the arteries. Infarcts are more likely to undergo hemorrhagic transformation (leaking of blood into the damaged area) than other types of ischemic stroke.

Intracerebral Hemorrhage

It generally occurs in small arteries or arterioles and is commonly due to hypertension, intracranial vascular malformations (including cavernous angiomas or arteriovenous malformations), cerebral amyloid angiopathy, or infarcts into which secondary hemorrhage has occurred. Other potential causes are trauma, bleeding disorders, amyloid angiopathy, illicit drug use (e.g., amphetamines or cocaine). The hematoma enlarges until pressure from surrounding tissue limits its growth, or until it decompresses by emptying into the ventricular system, CSF or the pial surface. A third of intracerebral bleed is into the brain's ventricles. ICH has a mortality rate of 44 percent after 30 days, higher than ischemic stroke or subarachnoid hemorrhage (which technically may also be classified as a type of stroke).

Other

Other causes may include spasm of an artery. This may occur due to cocaine.

Silent Stroke

A silent stroke is a stroke that does not have any outward symptoms, and the patients are typically unaware they have had a stroke. Despite not causing identifiable symptoms, a silent stroke still damages the brain, and places the patient at increased risk for both transient ischemic attack and major stroke in the future. Conversely, those who have had a major stroke are also at risk of having silent strokes. In a broad study in 1998, more than 11 million people were estimated to have experienced a stroke in the United States. Approximately 770,000 of these strokes were symptomatic and 11 million were first-ever silent MRI infarcts or hemorrhages. Silent strokes typically cause lesions which are detected via the use of neuroimaging such as MRI. Silent strokes are estimated to occur at five times the rate of symptomatic strokes. The risk of silent stroke increases with age, but may also affect younger adults and children, especially those with acute anemia.

Pathophysiology

Ischemic

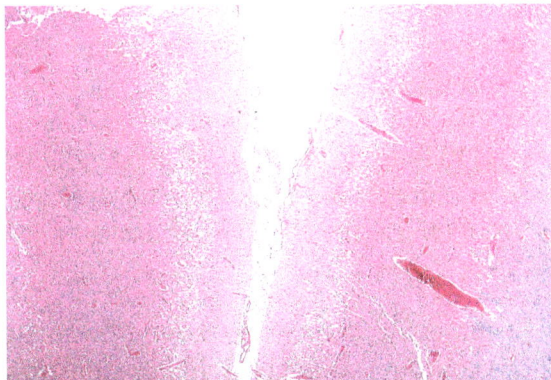

Micrograph showing cortical pseudolaminar necrosis, a finding seen in strokes on medical imaging and at autopsy. H&E-LFB stain.

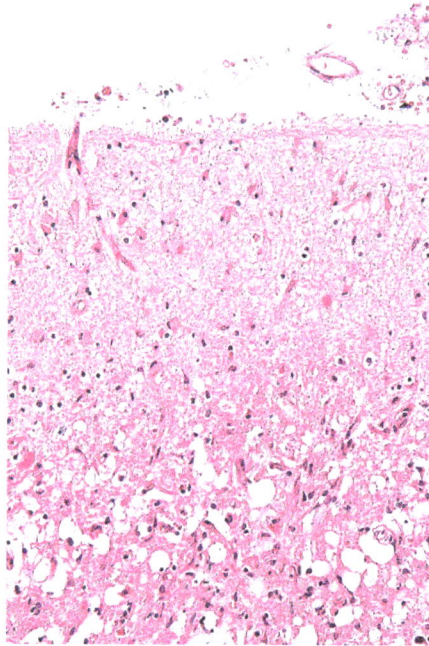

Micrograph of the superficial cerebral cortex showing neuron loss and reactive
astrocytes in a person that has had a stroke. H&E-LFB stain.

Ischemic stroke occurs because of a loss of blood supply to part of the brain, initiating
the ischemic cascade. Brain tissue ceases to function if deprived of oxygen for more
than 60 to 90 seconds, and after approximately three hours will suffer irreversible
injury possibly leading to the death of the tissue, i.e., infarction. (This is why fibrinolytics such as alteplase are given only until three hours since the onset of the stroke.)
Atherosclerosis may disrupt the blood supply by narrowing the lumen of blood vessels leading to a reduction of blood flow, by causing the formation of blood clots
within the vessel, or by releasing showers of small emboli through the disintegration
of atherosclerotic plaques. Embolic infarction occurs when emboli formed elsewhere
in the circulatory system, typically in the heart as a consequence of atrial fibrillation,
or in the carotid arteries, break off, enter the cerebral circulation, then lodge in and
block brain blood vessels. Since blood vessels in the brain are now blocked, the brain
becomes low in energy, and thus it resorts into using anaerobic metabolism within
the region of brain tissue affected by ischemia. Anaerobic metabolism produces less
adenosine triphosphate (ATP) but releases a by-product called lactic acid. Lactic acid
is an irritant which could potentially destroy cells since it is an acid and disrupts the
normal acid-base balance in the brain. The ischemia area is referred to as the "ischemic penumbra".

As oxygen or glucose becomes depleted in ischemic brain tissue, the production
of high energy phosphate compounds such as adenosine triphosphate (ATP) fails,
leading to failure of energy-dependent processes (such as ion pumping) necessary
for tissue cell survival. This sets off a series of interrelated events that result in

cellular injury and death. A major cause of neuronal injury is the release of the excitatory neurotransmitter glutamate. The concentration of glutamate outside the cells of the nervous system is normally kept low by so-called uptake carriers, which are powered by the concentration gradients of ions (mainly Na^+) across the cell membrane. However, stroke cuts off the supply of oxygen and glucose which powers the ion pumps maintaining these gradients. As a result, the transmembrane ion gradients run down, and glutamate transporters reverse their direction, releasing glutamate into the extracellular space. Glutamate acts on receptors in nerve cells (especially NMDA receptors), producing an influx of calcium which activates enzymes that digest the cells' proteins, lipids, and nuclear material. Calcium influx can also lead to the failure of mitochondria, which can lead further toward energy depletion and may trigger cell death due to programmed cell death.

Ischemia also induces production of oxygen free radicals and other reactive oxygen species. These react with and damage a number of cellular and extracellular elements. Damage to the blood vessel lining or endothelium is particularly important. In fact, many antioxidant neuroprotectants such as uric acid and NXY-059 work at the level of the endothelium and not in the brain *per se*. Free radicals also directly initiate elements of the programmed cell death cascade by means of redox signaling.

These processes are the same for any type of ischemic tissue and are referred to collectively as the *ischemic cascade*. However, brain tissue is especially vulnerable to ischemia since it has a little respiratory reserve and is completely dependent on aerobic metabolism, unlike most other organs.

In addition to damaging effects on brain cells, ischemia and infarction can result in loss of structural integrity of brain tissue and blood vessels, partly through the release of matrix metalloproteases, which are zinc- and calcium-dependent enzymes that break down collagen, hyaluronic acid, and other elements of connective tissue. Other proteases also contribute to this process. The loss of vascular structural integrity results in a breakdown of the protective blood brain barrier that contributes to cerebral edema, which can cause secondary progression of the brain injury.

Hemorrhagic

Hemorrhagic strokes are classified based on their underlying pathology. Some causes of hemorrhagic stroke are hypertensive hemorrhage, ruptured aneurysm, ruptured AV fistula, transformation of prior ischemic infarction, and drug induced bleeding. They result in tissue injury by causing compression of tissue from an expanding hematoma or hematomas. In addition, the pressure may lead to a loss of blood supply to affected tissue with resulting infarction, and the blood released by brain hemorrhage appears to have direct toxic effects on brain tissue and vasculature. Inflammation contributes to the secondary brain injury after hemorrhage.

Diagnosis

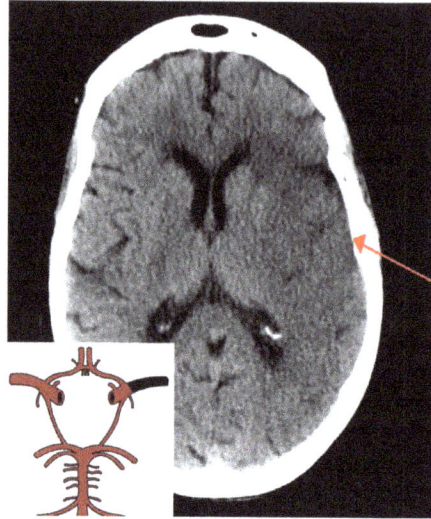

A CT showing early signs of a middle cerebral artery stroke with loss of definition
of the gyri and grey white boundary

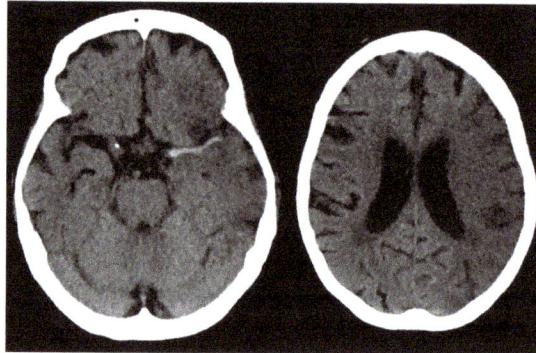

Dens media sign in a patient with middle cerebral artery infarction
shown on the left. Right image after 7 hours.

Stroke is diagnosed through several techniques: a neurological examination (such as
the NIHSS), CT scans (most often without contrast enhancements) or MRI scans, Dop-
pler ultrasound, and arteriography. The diagnosis of stroke itself is clinical, with assistance from the imaging techniques. Imaging techniques also assist in determining the
subtypes and cause of stroke. There is yet no commonly used blood test for the stroke
diagnosis itself, though blood tests may be of help in finding out the likely cause of
stroke.

Physical Examination

A physical examination, including taking a medical history of the symptoms and a neurological status, helps giving an evaluation of the location and severity of a stroke. It
can give a standard score on e.g., the NIH stroke scale.

Imaging

For diagnosing ischemic stroke in the emergency setting:

- CT scans (*without* contrast enhancements)

  sensitivity= 16%

  specificity= 96%

- MRI scan

  sensitivity= 83%

  specificity= 98%

For diagnosing hemorrhagic stroke in the emergency setting:

- CT scans (*without* contrast enhancements)

  sensitivity= 89%

  specificity= 100%

- MRI scan

  sensitivity= 81%

  specificity= 100%

For detecting chronic hemorrhages, MRI scan is more sensitive.

For the assessment of stable stroke, nuclear medicine scans SPECT and PET/CT may be helpful. SPECT documents cerebral blood flow and PET with FDG isotope the metabolic activity of the neurons.

Underlying Cause

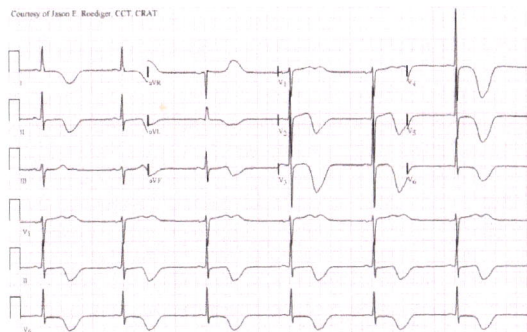

12-lead ECG of a patient with a stroke, showing large deeply inverted T-waves. Various ECG changes may occur in people with strokes and other brain disorders.

When a stroke has been diagnosed, various other studies may be performed to determine the underlying cause. With the current treatment and diagnosis options available, it is of particular importance to determine whether there is a peripheral source of emboli. Test selection may vary since the cause of stroke varies with age, comorbidity and the clinical presentation. The following are commonly used techniques:

- an ultrasound/doppler study of the carotid arteries (to detect carotid stenosis) or dissection of the precerebral arteries;

- an electrocardiogram (ECG) and echocardiogram (to identify arrhythmias and resultant clots in the heart which may spread to the brain vessels through the bloodstream);

- a Holter monitor study to identify intermittent abnormal heart rhythms;

- an angiogram of the cerebral vasculature (if a bleed is thought to have originated from an aneurysm or arteriovenous malformation);

- blood tests to determine if blood cholesterol is high, if there is an abnormal tendency to bleed, and if some rarer processes such as homocystinuria might be involved.

For hemorrhagic strokes, a CT or MRI scan with intravascular contrast may be able to identify abnormalities in the brain arteries (such as aneurysms) or other sources of bleeding, and structural MRI if this shows no cause. If this too does not identify an underlying reason for the bleeding, invasive cerebral angiography could be performed but this requires access to the bloodstream with an intravascular catheter and can cause further strokes as well as complications at the insertion site and this investigation is therefore reserved for specific situations. If there are symptoms suggesting that the hemorrhage might have occurred as a result of venous thrombosis, CT or MRI venography can be used to examine the cerebral veins.

Prevention

Given the disease burden of strokes, prevention is an important public health concern. Primary prevention is less effective than secondary prevention (as judged by the number needed to treat to prevent one stroke per year). Recent guidelines detail the evidence for primary prevention in stroke. In those who are otherwise healthy, aspirin does not appear beneficial and thus is not recommended. In people who have had a myocardial infarction or those with a high cardiovascular risk, it provides some protection against a first stroke. In those who have previously had a stroke, treatment with medications such as aspirin, clopidogrel, and dipyridamole may be beneficial. The U.S. Preventive Services Task Force (USPSTF) recommends against screening for carotid artery stenosis in those without symptoms.

Risk Factors

The most important modifiable risk factors for stroke are high blood pressure and atrial fibrillation although the size of the effect is small with 833 people have to be treated for 1 year to prevent one stroke. Other modifiable risk factors include high blood cholesterol levels, diabetes mellitus, cigarette smoking (active and passive), drinking lots of alcohol and drug use, lack of physical activity, obesity, processed red meat consumption and unhealthy diet. Alcohol use could predispose to ischemic stroke, and intracerebral and subarachnoid hemorrhage via multiple mechanisms (for example via hypertension, atrial fibrillation, rebound thrombocytosis and platelet aggregation and clotting disturbances). Drugs, most commonly amphetamines and cocaine, can induce stroke through damage to the blood vessels in the brain and/or acute hypertension.

High levels of physical activity reduce the risk of stroke by about 26%. There is a lack of high quality studies looking at promotional efforts to improve lifestyle factors. Nonetheless, given the large body of circumstantial evidence, best medical management for stroke includes advice on diet, exercise, smoking and alcohol use. Medication is the most common method of stroke prevention; carotid endarterectomy can be a useful surgical method of preventing stroke.

Blood Pressure

High blood pressure accounts for 35–50% of stroke risk. Blood pressure reduction of 10 mmHg systolic or 5 mmHg diastolic reduces the risk of stroke by ~40%. Lowering blood pressure has been conclusively shown to prevent both ischemic and hemorrhagic strokes. It is equally important in secondary prevention. Even patients older than 80 years and those with isolated systolic hypertension benefit from antihypertensive therapy. The available evidence does not show large differences in stroke prevention between antihypertensive drugs —therefore, other factors such as protection against other forms of cardiovascular disease and cost should be considered. The routine use of beta-blockers following a stroke or TIA has not been shown to result in benefits.

Blood Lipids

High cholesterol levels have been inconsistently associated with (ischemic) stroke. Statins have been shown to reduce the risk of stroke by about 15%. Since earlier meta-analyses of other lipid-lowering drugs did not show a decreased risk, statins might exert their effect through mechanisms other than their lipid-lowering effects.

Diabetes Mellitus

Diabetes mellitus increases the risk of stroke by 2 to 3 times. While intensive blood sugar control has been shown to reduce small blood vessel complications such as kidney damage and damage to the retina of the eye it has not been shown to reduce large blood vessel complications such as stroke.

Anticoagulation Drugs

Oral anticoagulants such as warfarin have been the mainstay of stroke prevention for over 50 years. However, several studies have shown that aspirin and antiplatelet drugs are highly effective in secondary prevention after a stroke or transient ischemic attack. Low doses of aspirin (for example 75–150 mg) are as effective as high doses but have fewer side effects; the lowest effective dose remains unknown. Thienopyridines (clopidogrel, ticlopidine) might be slightly more effective than aspirin and have a decreased risk of gastrointestinal bleeding, but are more expensive. Clopidogrel has less side effects than ticlopidine. Dipyridamole can be added to aspirin therapy to provide a small additional benefit, even though headache is a common side effect. Low-dose aspirin is also effective for stroke prevention after having a myocardial infarction.

Those with atrial fibrillation have a 5% a year risk of stroke, and this risk is higher in those with valvular atrial fibrillation. Depending on the stroke risk, anticoagulation with medications such as warfarin or aspirin is useful for prevention. Except in people with atrial fibrillation, oral anticoagulants are not advised for stroke prevention —any benefit is offset by bleeding risk.

In primary prevention however, antiplatelet drugs did not reduce the risk of ischemic stroke but increased the risk of major bleeding. Further studies are needed to investigate a possible protective effect of aspirin against ischemic stroke in women.

Surgery

Carotid endarterectomy or carotid angioplasty can be used to remove atherosclerotic narrowing of the carotid artery. There is evidence supporting this procedure in selected cases. Endarterectomy for a significant stenosis has been shown to be useful in preventing further strokes in those who have already had one. Carotid artery stenting has not been shown to be equally useful. People are selected for surgery based on age, gender, degree of stenosis, time since symptoms and the person's preferences. Surgery is most efficient when not delayed too long —the risk of recurrent stroke in a patient who has a 50% or greater stenosis is up to 20% after 5 years, but endarterectomy reduces this risk to around 5%. The number of procedures needed to cure one patient was 5 for early surgery (within two weeks after the initial stroke), but 125 if delayed longer than 12 weeks.

Screening for carotid artery narrowing has not been shown to be a useful test in the general population. Studies of surgical intervention for carotid artery stenosis without symptoms have shown only a small decrease in the risk of stroke. To be beneficial, the complication rate of the surgery should be kept below 4%. Even then, for 100 surgeries, 5 patients will benefit by avoiding stroke, 3 will develop stroke despite surgery, 3 will develop stroke or die due to the surgery itself, and 89 will remain stroke-free but would also have done so without intervention.

Diet

Nutrition, specifically the Mediterranean-style diet, has the potential for decreasing the risk of having a stroke by more than half. It does not appear that lowering levels of homocysteine with folic acid affects the risk of stroke.

Women

A number of specific recommendations have been made for women including taking aspirin after the 11th week of pregnancy if there is a history of previous chronic high blood pressure and taking blood pressure medications during pregnancy if the blood pressure is greater than 150 mmHg systolic or greater than 100 mmHg diastolic. In those who have previously had preeclampsia other risk factors should be treated more aggressively.

Previous Stroke or TIA

Keeping blood pressure below 140/90 mmHg is recommended. Anticoagulation can prevent recurrent ischemic strokes. Among people with nonvalvular atrial fibrillation, anticoagulation can reduce stroke by 60% while antiplatelet agents can reduce stroke by 20%. However, a recent meta-analysis suggests harm from anticoagulation started early after an embolic stroke. Stroke prevention treatment for atrial fibrillation is determined according to the CHA2DS2–VASc score. The most widely used anticoagulant to prevent thromboembolic stroke in patients with nonvalvular atrial fibrillation is the oral agent warfarin while a number of newer agents including dabigatran are alternatives which do not require prothrombin time monitoring.

Anticoagulants, when used following stroke, should not be stopped for dental procedures.

If studies show carotid artery stenosis, and the person has a degree of residual function on the affected side, carotid endarterectomy (surgical removal of the stenosis) may decrease the risk of recurrence if performed rapidly after stroke.

Management

Ischemic Stroke

Aspirin reduces the overall risk of recurrence by 13% with greater benefit early on. Definitive therapy within the first few hours is aimed at removing the blockage by breaking the clot down (thrombolysis), or by removing it mechanically (thrombectomy). The philosophical premise underlying the importance of rapid stroke intervention was summed up as *Time is Brain!* in the early 1990s. Years later, that same idea, that rapid cerebral blood flow restoration results in fewer brain cells dying, has been proved and quantified.

Tight blood sugar control in the first few hours does not improve outcomes and may cause harm. High blood pressure is also not typically lowered as this has not been found to be helpful. Cerebrolysin, a mix of pig brain tissue used to treat acute ischemic stroke in many Asian and European countries, does not improve outcomes and may increase the risk of severe adverse events.

Thrombolysis

Thrombolysis, such as with recombinant tissue plasminogen activator (rtPA), in acute ischemic stroke, when given within three hours of symptom onset results in an overall benefit of 10% with respect to living without disability. It does not, however, improve chances of survival. Benefit is greater the earlier it is used. Between three and four and a half hours the effects are less clear. A 2014 review found a 5% increase in the number of people living without disability at three to six months; however, there was a 2% increased risk of death in the short term. After four and a half hours thrombolysis worsens outcomes. These benefits or lack of benefits occurred regardless of the age of the person treated. There is no reliable way to determine who will have an intracranial bleed post-treatment versus who will not.

Its use is endorsed by the American Heart Association and the American Academy of Neurology as the recommended treatment for acute stroke within three hours of onset of symptoms as long as there are not other contraindications (such as abnormal lab values, high blood pressure, or recent surgery). This position for tPA is based upon the findings of two studies by one group of investigators which showed that tPA improves the chances for a good neurological outcome. When administered within the first three hours thrombolysis improves functional outcome without affecting mortality. 6.4% of people with large strokes developed substantial brain bleeding as a complication from being given tPA thus part of the reason for increased short term mortality. Additionally, the American Academy of Emergency Medicine states that objective evidence regarding the efficacy, safety, and applicability of tPA for acute ischemic stroke is insufficient to warrant its classification as standard of care. Intra-arterial fibrinolysis, where a catheter is passed up an artery into the brain and the medication is injected at the site of thrombosis, has been found to improve outcomes in people with acute ischemic stroke.

Surgery

Surgical removal of the blood clot causing the ischemic stroke may improve outcomes if done within 7 hours of the start of symptoms in those with an anterior circulation large artery clot. It however does not change the risk of death.

Strokes affecting large portions of the brain can cause significant brain swelling with secondary brain injury in surrounding tissue. This phenomenon is mainly encountered in strokes affecting brain tissue dependent upon the middle cerebral artery for blood supply and is also called "malignant cerebral infarction" because it carries a dismal prognosis. Relief of the pressure may be attempted with medication, but some require hemicraniectomy, the temporary surgical removal of the skull on one side of the head. This decreases the risk of death, although some more people survive with disability who would otherwise have died.

Hemorrhagic Stroke

People with intracerebral hemorrhage require supportive care, including blood pressure control if required. People are monitored for changes in the level of consciousness, and their blood sugar and oxygenation are kept at optimum levels. Anticoagulants and antithrombotics can make bleeding worse and are generally discontinued (and reversed if possible). A proportion may benefit from neurosurgical intervention to remove the blood and treat the underlying cause, but this depends on the location and the size of the hemorrhage as well as patient-related factors, and ongoing research is being conducted into the question as to which people with intracerebral hemorrhage may benefit.

In subarachnoid hemorrhage, early treatment for underlying cerebral aneurysms may reduce the risk of further hemorrhages. Depending on the site of the aneurysm this may be by surgery that involves opening the skull or endovascularly (through the blood vessels).

Stroke Unit

Ideally, people who have had a stroke are admitted to a "stroke unit", a ward or dedicated area in a hospital staffed by nurses and therapists with experience in stroke treatment. It has been shown that people admitted to a stroke unit have a higher chance of surviving than those admitted elsewhere in hospital, even if they are being cared for by doctors without experience in stroke.

Rehabilitation

Stroke rehabilitation is the process by which those with disabling strokes undergo treatment to help them return to normal life as much as possible by regaining and relearning the skills of everyday living. It also aims to help the survivor understand and adapt to difficulties, prevent secondary complications and educate family members to play a supporting role.

A rehabilitation team is usually multidisciplinary as it involves staff with different skills working together to help the patient. These include physicians trained in rehabilitation medicine, clinical pharmacists, nursing staff, physiotherapists, occupational thera-pists, speech and language therapists, and orthotists. Some teams may also include psychologists and social workers, since at least one-third of affected people manifests post stroke depression. Validated instruments such as the Barthel scale may be used to assess the likelihood of a stroke patient being able to manage at home with or without support subsequent to discharge from a hospital.

Good nursing care is fundamental in maintaining skin care, feeding, hydration, po-sitioning, and monitoring vital signs such as temperature, pulse, and blood pressure. Stroke rehabilitation begins almost immediately.

For most people with stroke, physical therapy (PT), occupational therapy (OT) and speech-language pathology (SLP) are the cornerstones of the rehabilitation process. Often, assistive technology such as wheelchairs, walkers and canes may be beneficial. Many mobility problems can be improved by the use of ankle foot orthoses. PT and OT have overlapping areas of expertise; however, PT focuses on joint range of motion and strength by performing exercises and relearning functional tasks such as bed mobility, transferring, walking and other gross motor functions. Physiotherapists can also work with patients to improve awareness and use of the hemiplegic side. Rehabilitation in-volves working on the ability to produce strong movements or the ability to perform tasks using normal patterns. Emphasis is often concentrated on functional tasks and patient's goals. One example physiotherapists employ to promote motor learning in-volves constraint-induced movement therapy. Through continuous practice the patient relearns to use and adapt the hemiplegic limb during functional activities to create lasting permanent changes. OT is involved in training to help relearn everyday activi-ties known as the activities of daily living (ADLs) such as eating, drinking, dressing, bathing, cooking, reading and writing, and toileting. Speech and language therapy is appropriate for people with the speech production disorders: dysarthria and apraxia of speech, aphasia, cognitive-communication impairments and/or problems with swal-lowing.

Patients may have particular problems, such as dysphagia, which can cause swallowed material to pass into the lungs and cause aspiration pneumonia. The condition may improve with time, but in the interim, a nasogastric tube may be inserted, enabling liquid food to be given directly into the stomach. If swallowing is still deemed unsafe, then a percutaneous endoscopic gastrostomy (PEG) tube is passed and this can remain indefinitely.

Treatment of spasticity related to stroke often involves early mobilizations, commonly performed by a physiotherapist, combined with elongation of spastic muscles and sus-tained stretching through various positionings. Gaining initial improvement in range of motion is often achieved through rhythmic rotational patterns associated with the affected limb. After full range has been achieved by the therapist, the limb should be positioned in the lengthened positions to prevent against further contractures, skin breakdown, and disuse of the limb with the use of splints or other tools to stabilize the joint. Cold in the form of ice wraps or ice packs have been proven to briefly reduce spasticity by temporarily dampening neural firing rates. Electrical stimulation to the antagonist muscles or vibrations has also been used with some success.

Stroke rehabilitation should be started as quickly as possible and can last anywhere from a few days to over a year. Most return of function is seen in the first few months, and then improvement falls off with the "window" considered officially by U.S. state rehabilitation units and others to be closed after six months, with little chance of further improvement. However, patients have been known to continue to improve for years, regaining and strengthening abilities like writing, walking, running, and talking. Daily rehabilitation exercises should continue to be part of the stroke patient's routine. Complete recovery is unusual but not impossible and most patients will improve to some extent: proper diet and exercise are known to help the brain to recover.

Some current and future therapy methods include the use of virtual reality and video games for rehabilitation. These forms of rehabilitation offer potential for motivating patients to perform specific therapy tasks that many other forms do not. Many clinics and hospitals are adopting the use of these off-the-shelf devices for exercise, social interaction, and rehabilitation because they are affordable, accessible and can be used within the clinic and home.

Other novel non-invasive rehabilitation methods are currently being developed to augment physical therapy to improve motor function of stroke patients, such as transcranial magnetic stimulation (TMS) and transcranial direct-current stimulation (tDCS) and robotic therapies.

A stroke can also reduce people's general fitness. Reduced fitness can reduce capacity for rehabilitation as well as general health. A systematic review found that there are inadequate long-term data about the effects of exercise and training on death, dependence and disability after a stroke. However, cardiorespiratory training added to walking programs in rehabilitation can improve speed, tolerance and independence during walking.

The ability to walk independently in their community, indoors or outdoors, is important following stroke. Although no negative effects have been reported, it is unclear if outcomes can improve with these walking programs when compared to usual treatment.

Self-management

A stroke can affect the ability to live independently and with quality. Self-management programs are a special training that educates stroke survivors about stroke and its consequences, helps them acquire skills to cope with their challenges, and helps them set and meet their own goals during their recovery process. These programs are tailored to the target audience, and lead by someone trained and expert in stroke and its consequences (most commonly professionals, but also stroke survivors and peers). A 2016 review reported that these programs improve the quality of life after stroke, without negative effects. People with stroke felt more empowered, happy and satisfied with life after participating in this training.

Prognosis

Disability affects 75% of stroke survivors enough to decrease their employability. Stroke can affect people physically, mentally, emotionally, or a combination of the three. The results of stroke vary widely depending on size and location of the lesion. Dysfunctions correspond to areas in the brain that have been damaged.

Some of the physical disabilities that can result from stroke include muscle weakness, numbness, pressure sores, pneumonia, incontinence, apraxia (inability to perform learned movements), difficulties carrying out daily activities, appetite loss, speech loss, vision loss and pain. If the stroke is severe enough, or in a certain location such as parts of the brainstem, coma or death can result.

Emotional problems following a stroke can be due to direct damage to emotional centers in the brain or from frustration and difficulty adapting to new limitations. Post-stroke emotional difficulties include anxiety, panic attacks, flat affect (failure to express emotions), mania, apathy and psychosis. Other difficulties may include a decreased ability to communicate emotions through facial expression, body language and voice.

Disruption in self-identity, relationships with others, and emotional well-being can lead to social consequences after stroke due to the lack of ability to communicate. Many people who experience communication impairments after a stroke find it more difficult to cope with the social issues rather than physical impairments. Broader aspects of care must address the emotional impact speech impairment has on those who experience difficulties with speech after a stroke. Those who experience a stroke are at risk of paralysis which could result in a self disturbed body image which may also lead to other social issues.

30 to 50% of stroke survivors suffer post-stroke depression, which is characterized by lethargy, irritability, sleep disturbances, lowered self-esteem and withdrawal. Depression can reduce motivation and worsen outcome, but can be treated with social and family support, psychotherapy and, in severe cases, antidepressants.

Emotional lability, another consequence of stroke, causes the person to switch quickly between emotional highs and lows and to express emotions inappropriately, for instance with an excess of laughing or crying with little or no provocation. While these expressions of emotion usually correspond to the person's actual emotions, a more severe form of emotional lability causes the affected person to laugh and cry pathologically, without regard to context or emotion. Some people show the opposite of what they feel, for example crying when they are happy. Emotional lability occurs in about 20% of those who have had a stroke. Those with a right hemisphere stroke are more likely to have an empathy problems which can make communication harder.

Cognitive deficits resulting from stroke include perceptual disorders, aphasia, dementia, and problems with attention and memory. A stroke sufferer may be unaware of his or her own disabilities, a condition called anosognosia. In a condition called hemispatial neglect, the affected person is unable to attend to anything on the side of space opposite to the damaged hemisphere.

Cognitive and psychological outcome after a stroke can be affected by the age at which the stroke happened, pre-stroke baseline intellectual functioning, psychiatric history and whether there is pre-existing brain pathology.

Up to 10% of people following a stroke develop seizures, most commonly in the week subsequent to the event; the severity of the stroke increases the likelihood of a seizure.

Epidemiology

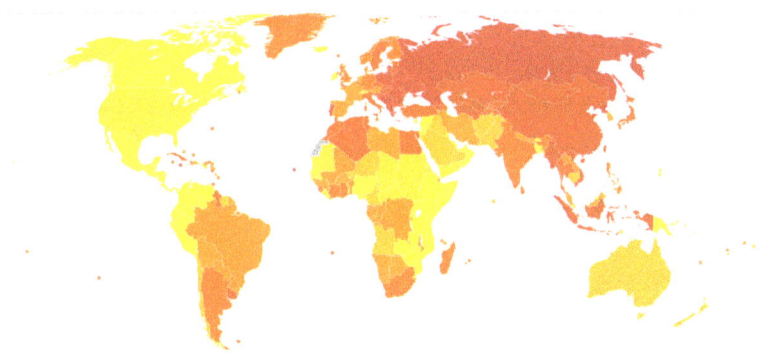

Stroke deaths per million persons in 2012

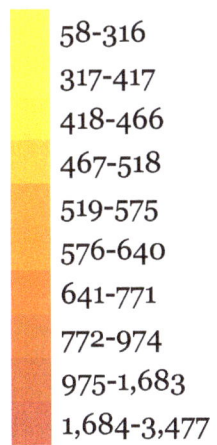

	58-316
	317-417
	418-466
	467-518
	519-575
	576-640
	641-771
	772-974
	975-1,683
	1,684-3,477

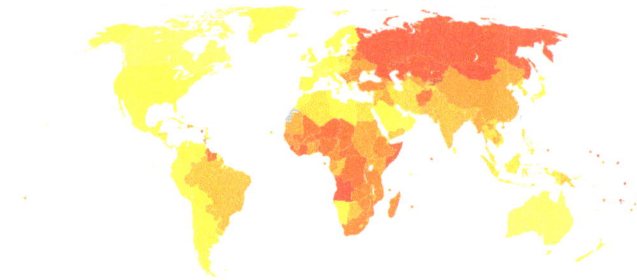

Disability-adjusted life year for cerebral vascular disease per 100,000 inhabitants in 2004.

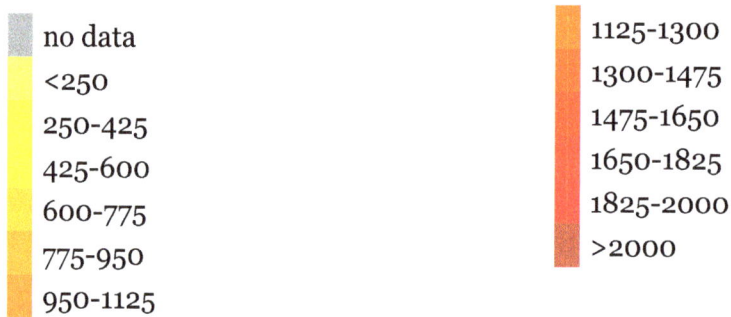

no data		1125-1300	
<250		1300-1475	
250-425		1475-1650	
425-600		1650-1825	
600-775		1825-2000	
775-950		>2000	
950-1125			

Stroke was the second most frequent cause of death worldwide in 2011, accounting for 6.2 million deaths (~11% of the total). Approximately 17 million people had a stroke in 2010 and 33 million people have previously had a stroke and were still alive. Between 1990 and 2010 the number of strokes decreased by approximately 10% in the developed world and increased by 10% in the developing world. Overall, two-thirds of strokes occurred in those over 65 years old. South Asians are at particularly high risk of stroke, accounting for 40% of global stroke deaths.

It is ranked after heart disease and before cancer. In the United States stroke is a leading cause of disability, and recently declined from the third leading to the fourth leading cause of death. Geographic disparities in stroke incidence have been observed, including the existence of a "stroke belt" in the southeastern United States, but causes of these disparities have not been explained.

The risk of stroke increases exponentially from 30 years of age, and the cause varies by age. Advanced age is one of the most significant stroke risk factors. 95% of strokes occur in people age 45 and older, and two-thirds of strokes occur in those over the age of 65. A person's risk of dying if he or she does have a stroke also increases with age. However, stroke can occur at any age, including in childhood.

Family members may have a genetic tendency for stroke or share a lifestyle that contributes to stroke. Higher levels of Von Willebrand factor are more common amongst people who have had ischemic stroke for the first time. The results of this study found that the only significant genetic factor was the person's blood type. Having had a stroke in the past greatly increases one's risk of future strokes.

Men are 25% more likely to suffer strokes than women, yet 60% of deaths from stroke occur in women. Since women live longer, they are older on average when they have their strokes and thus more often killed. Some risk factors for stroke apply only to women. Primary among these are pregnancy, childbirth, menopause, and the treatment thereof (HRT).

History

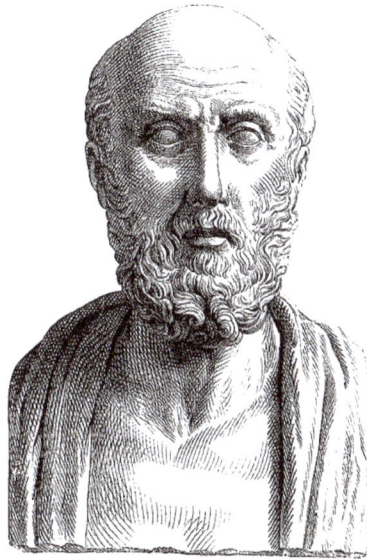

Hippocrates first described the sudden paralysis that is often associated with stroke.

Episodes of stroke and familial stroke have been reported from the 2nd millennium BC onward in ancient Mesopotamia and Persia. Hippocrates (460 to 370 BC) was first to describe the phenomenon of sudden paralysis that is often associated with ischemia. Apoplexy, from the Greek word meaning "struck down with violence", first appeared in Hippocratic writings to describe this phenomenon. The word *stroke* was used as a synonym for apoplectic seizure as early as 1599, and is a fairly literal translation of the Greek term.

In 1658, in his *Apoplexia*, Johann Jacob Wepfer (1620–1695) identified the cause of hemorrhagic stroke when he suggested that people who had died of apoplexy had bleeding in their brains. Wepfer also identified the main arteries supplying the brain, the vertebral and carotid arteries, and identified the cause of a type of ischemic stroke known as a cerebral infarction when he suggested that apoplexy might be caused by a blockage to those vessels. Rudolf Virchow first described the mechanism of thromboembolism as a major factor.

The term *cerebrovascular accident* was introduced in 1927, reflecting a "growing awareness and acceptance of vascular theories and (...) recognition of the consequences of a sudden disruption in the vascular supply of the brain". Its use is now discouraged by a number of neurology textbooks, reasoning that the connotation of fortuitousness carried by the word *accident* insufficiently highlights the modifiability of the underlying risk factors. *Cerebrovascular insult* may be used interchangeably.

The term *brain attack* was introduced for use to underline the acute nature of stroke according to the American Stroke Association, who since 1990 have used the term, and is used colloquially to refer to both ischemic as well as hemorrhagic stroke.

Research

Angioplasty and Stenting

Angioplasty and stenting have begun to be looked at as possible viable options in treatment of acute ischemic stroke. Intra-cranial stenting in symptomatic intracranial arterial stenosis, the rate of technical success (reduction to stenosis of <50%) ranged from 90-98%, and the rate of major peri-procedural complications ranged from 4-10%. The rates of restenosis and/or stroke following the treatment were also favorable. This data suggests that a randomized controlled trial is needed to more completely evaluate the possible therapeutic advantage of this preventative measure.

Mechanical Thrombectomy

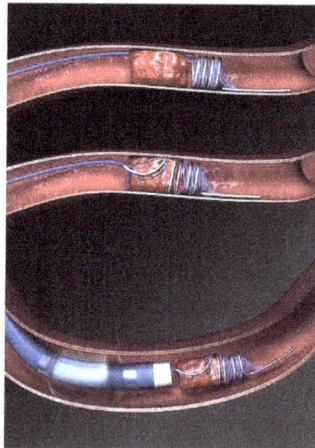

MERCI Retriever L5.

Removal of the clot may be attempted in those where it occurs within a large blood vessel and may be an option for those who either are not eligible for or do not improve with intravenous thrombolytics. Significant complications occur in about 7%.

Neuroprotection

Neuroprotective agents including antioxidants which combat reactive oxygen species, or inhibit programmed cell death, or inhibit excitatory neurotransmitters have been shown experimentally to reduce tissue injury caused by ischemia. Until recently, human clinical trials with neuroprotective agents have failed, with the probable exception of deep barbiturate-induced coma. Disufenton sodium, the disulfonyl derivative of the radical-scavenging phenylbutylnitrone, was reported to be neuroprotective. This agent is thought to work at the level of the blood vessel lining. However the favourable results evidenced from one large-scale trial were not reproduced in a second trial. So that the benefit of disufenton sodium is questionable.

Hyperbaric oxygen therapy has been studied as a possible protective measure, but as of 2014, while the benefits of this have not been ruled out, further research is said to be needed.

Brain Ischemia

Brain ischemia (a.k.a. cerebral ischemia, cerebrovascular ischemia) is a condition in which there is insufficient blood flow to the brain to meet metabolic demand. This leads to poor oxygen supply or cerebral hypoxia and thus to the death of brain tissue or cerebral infarction / ischemic stroke. It is a sub-type of stroke along with subarachnoid hemorrhage and intracerebral hemorrhage.

Ischemia leads to alterations in brain metabolism, reduction in metabolic rates, and energy crisis.

There are two types of ischemia: focal ischemia, which is confined to a specific region of the brain; and global ischemia, which encompasses wide areas of brain tissue.

The main symptoms involve impairments in vision, body movement, and speaking. The causes of brain ischemia vary from sickle cell anemia to congenital heart defects. Symptoms of brain ischemia can include unconsciousness, blindness, problems with coordination, and weakness in the body. Other effects that may result from brain ischemia are stroke, cardiorespiratory arrest, and irreversible brain damage.

An interruption of blood flow to the brain for more than 10 seconds causes unconsciousness, and an interruption in flow for more than a few minutes generally results in irreversible brain damage. In 1974, Hossmann and Zimmermann demonstrated that ischemia induced in mammalian brains for up to an hour can be at least partially recovered. Accordingly, this discovery raised the possibility of intervening after brain ischemia before the damage becomes irreversible.

Classification

The broad term, "stroke" can be divided into three categories: brain ischemia, subarachnoid hemorrhage and intracerebral hemorrhage. Brain ischemia can be further subdivided, by cause, into thrombotic, embolic, and hypoperfusion. Thrombotic and embolic are generally focal or multifocal in nature while hypoperfusion affects the brain globally.

Focal Brain Ischemia

Focal brain ischemia occurs when a blood clot has occluded a cerebral vessel. Focal brain ischemia reduces blood flow to a specific brain region, increasing the risk of cell death to that particular area. It can be either caused by thrombosis or embolism.

Global Brain Ischemia

Global brain ischemia occurs when blood flow to the brain is halted or drastically reduced. This is commonly caused by cardiac arrest. If sufficient circulation is restored within a short period of time, symptoms may be transient. However, if a significant amount of time passes before restoration, brain damage may be permanent. While reperfusion may be essential to protecting as much brain tissue as possible, it may also lead to reperfusion injury. Reperfusion injury is classified as the damage that ensues after restoration of blood supply to ischemic tissue.

Symptoms

The symptoms of brain ischemia reflect the anatomical region undergoing blood and oxygen deprivation. Ischemia within the arteries branching from the internal carotid artery may result in symptoms such as blindness in one eye, weakness in one arm or leg, or weakness in one entire side of the body. Ischemia within the arteries branching from the vertebral arteries in the back of the brain may result in symptoms such as dizziness, vertigo, double vision, or weakness on both sides of the body. Other symptoms include difficulty speaking, slurred speech, and the loss of coordination. The symptoms of brain ischemia range from mild to severe. Further, symptoms can last from a few seconds to a few minutes or extended periods of time. If the brain becomes damaged irreversibly and infarction occurs, the symptoms may be permanent.

Similar to cerebral hypoxia, severe or prolonged brain ischemia will result in unconsciousness, brain damage or death, mediated by the ischemic cascade.

Multiple cerebral ischemic events may lead to subcortical ischemic depression, also known as vascular depression. This condition is most commonly seen in elderly depressed patients. Late onset depression is increasingly seen as a distinct sub-type of depression, and can be detected with an MRI.

Causes

Brain ischemia has been linked to a variety of diseases or abnormalities. Individuals with sickle cell anemia, compressed blood vessels, ventricular tachycardia, plaque buildup in the arteries, blood clots, extremely low blood pressure as a result of heart attack, and congenital heart defects have a higher predisposition to brain ischemia in comparison their healthy counterparts.

Sickle cell anemia may cause brain ischemia associated with the irregularly shaped blood cells. Sickle shaped blood cells clot more easily than normal blood cells, impeding blood flow to the brain.

Compression of blood vessels may also lead to brain ischemia, by blocking the arteries that carry oxygen to the brain. Tumors are one cause of blood vessel compression.

Ventricular tachycardia represents a series of irregular heartbeats that may cause the heart to completely shut down resulting in cessation of oxygen flow. Further, irregular heartbeats may result in formation of blood clots, thus leading to oxygen deprivation to all organs.

Blockage of arteries due to plaque buildup may also result in ischemia. Even a small amount of plaque build up can result in the narrowing of passageways, causing that area to become more prone to blood clots. Large blood clots can also cause ischemia by blocking blood flow.

A heart attack can also cause brain ischemia due to the correlation that exists between heart attack and low blood pressure. Extremely low blood pressure usually represents the inadequate oxygenation of tissues. Untreated heart attacks may slow blood flow enough that blood may start to clot and prevent the flow of blood to the brain or other major organs. Extremely low blood pressure can also result from drug overdose and reactions to drugs. Therefore, brain ischemia can result from events other than heart attacks.

Congenital heart defects may also cause brain ischemia due to the lack of appropriate artery formation and connection. People with congenital heart defects may also be prone to blood clots.

Other pathological events that may result in brain ischemia include cardiorespiratory arrest, stroke, and severe irreversible brain damage.

Recently, Moyamoya disease has also been identified as a potential cause for brain ischemia. Moyamoya disease is an extremely rare cerebrovascular condition that limits blood circulation to the brain, consequently leading to oxygen deprivation.

Pathophysiology

During brain ischemia, the brain cannot perform aerobic metabolism due to the loss of oxygen and substrate. The brain is not able to switch to anaerobic metabolism and because it does not have any long term energy stored the levels of adenosine triphosphate (ATP) drop rapidly and approach zero within 4 minutes. In the absence of biochemical energy, cells begin to lose the ability to maintain electrochemical gradients. Consequently, there is a massive influx of calcium into the cytosol, a massive release of glutamate from synaptic vesicles, lipolysis, calpain activation, and the arrest of protein synthesis. Additionally, removal of metabolic wastes is slowed. The interruption of blood flow to the brain for ten seconds results in the immediate loss of consciousness. The interruption of blood flow for twenty seconds results in the stopping of electrical activity. An area called a penumbra, may result, wherein neurons do not receive enough blood to communicate, however do receive sufficient oxygenation to avoid cell death for a short period of time.

Treatment

Alteplase (tpa) is an effective medication for acute ischemic stroke. When given within 3 hours, treatment with tpa significantly improves the probability of a favourable out-come versus treatment with placebo.

The outcome of brain ischemia is influenced by the quality of subsequent supportive care. Systemic blood pressure (or slightly above) should be maintained so that cere-bral blood flow is restored. Also, hypoxaemia and hypercapnia should be avoided. Sei-zures can induce more damage; accordingly, anticonvulsants should be prescribed and should a seizure occur, aggressive treatment should be undertaken. Hyperglycaemia should also be avoided during brain ischemia.

Management

When someone presents with an ischemic event, treatment of the underlying cause is critical for prevention of further episodes.

Anticoagulation with warfarin or heparin may be used if the patient has atrial fibrilla-tion.

Operative procedures such as carotid endarterectomy and carotid stenting may be per-formed if the patient has a significant amount of plaque in the carotid arteries associat-ed with the local ischemic events.

Research

Therapeutic hypothermia has been attempted to improve results post brain ischemia. This procedure was suggested to be beneficial based on its effects post cardiac arrest. Evidence supporting the use of therapeutic hypothermia after brain ischemia, however, is limited.

A closely related disease to brain ischemia is brain hypoxia. Brain hypoxia is the condi-tion in which there is a decrease in the oxygen supply to the brain even in the presence of adequate blood flow. If hypoxia lasts for long periods of time, coma, seizures, and even brain death may occur. Symptoms of brain hypoxia are similar to ischemia and include inattentiveness, poor judgment, memory loss, and a decrease in motor coordi-nation. Potential causes of brain hypoxia are suffocation, carbon monoxide poisoning, severe anemia, and use of drugs such as cocaine and other amphetamines. Other causes associated with brain hypoxia include drowning, strangling, choking, cardiac arrest, head trauma, and complications during general anesthesia. Treatment strategies for brain hypoxia vary depending on the original cause of injury.

Brainstem Stroke Syndrome

A brainstem stroke syndrome is a condition involving a stroke of the brainstem. Because of their location, they often involve impairment both of the cranial nuclei and of the long tracts. A person may have vertigo, dizziness and severe imbalance without the hallmark of most strokes – weakness on one side of the body. The symptoms of vertigo, dizziness or imbalance usually occur together; dizziness alone is not a sign of stroke. Brainstem stroke can also cause diplopia, slurred speech and decreased level of consciousness. A more serious outcome is locked-in syndrome.

Notable Cases

Kate Allatt

Kate Allatt is a mother-of-three from Sheffield, South Yorkshire. She has successfully recovered from locked-in syndrome. Now she runs *Fighting Strokes*, and devotes her life to assisting those with locked-in syndrome.

Jean-Dominique Bauby

Parisian journalist Jean-Dominique Bauby suffered a stroke in December 1995, and, when he awoke 20 days later, he found his body was almost completely paralyzed; he could control only his left eyelid. By blinking this eye, he slowly dictated one alphabetic character at a time and, in so doing, was able over a great deal of time to write his memoir, *The Diving Bell and the Butterfly*. Three days after it was published in March 1997, Bauby died of pneumonia. The 2007 film *The Diving Bell and the Butterfly* is a screen adaptation of Bauby's memoir. Jean-Dominique was instrumental in forming the *Association du Locked-In Syndrome* (ALIS) in France.

Rabbi Ronnie Cahana

In the summer of 2011, Rabbi Ronnie Cahana, Rabbi Emeritus of Congregation Beth-El in Montreal, suffered a severe brainstem stroke that left him in a locked-in state, able to communicate only with his eyes. With the help of his family, he continued to write poems and sermons for his congregation, letter by letter, through blinking. He has since regained his ability to breathe by himself and speak with his mouth. He describes his experiences as a blessing and a spiritual revelation of body and mind. His story was told in a Ted talk given by his daughter called: "My Father, Locked-in his Body but Soaring Free". He is the son of painter Alice Lok Cahana.

Tony Nicklinson

Tony Nicklinson, of Melksham, Wiltshire, England, was left paralysed after suffering a stroke in June 2005, at age 51. In the years that followed, he started a legal battle for a right to assisted death. On 16 August 2012, his request was turned down by the High Court of Justice. On learning the outcome of his appeal, he refused to eat, contracted pneumonia, deteriorated rapidly and died a week later on 22 August 2012, aged 58.

Julia Tavalaro

In 1966, Julia Tavalaro, then aged 32, suffered two strokes and a brain hemorrhage and was sent to Goldwater Memorial Hospital on Roosevelt Island, New York. For six years, she was believed to be in a vegetative state. In 1972, a family member noticed her trying to smile after she heard a joke. After alerting doctors, a speech therapist, Arlene Kratt, discerned cognizance in her eye movements. Kratt and an occupational therapist, Joyce Sabari, were eventually able to convince doctors she was in a locked-in state. After learning to communicate with eye blinks in response to letters being pointed to on an alphabet board, she became a poet and author. Eventually, she gained the ability to move her head enough to touch a switch with her cheek, which operated a motorized wheelchair and a computer. She gained national attention in 1995 when the Richard E. Meyer of the *Los Angeles Times* published a cover story about Tavalaro. In 1997, Erika Duncan's profile of Julia and her co-author Richard Tayson, "Decades After Silence, a Voice Is Recognized," ran in the Long Island edition of *The New York Times* and in April 1997, "The Long Road Home" appeared in *Newsday*. Julia Tavalaro appears with Richard Tayson on Dateline NBC and Melissa Etheridge's Beyond Chance (Lifetime). Their book was published by Viking-Penguin in 1998 and was translated into German, where it was published as *Bis auf den Grund des Ozeans* by Verlag Herder. Tavalaro's story became a bestseller in Germany. She died in 2003 at the age of 68.

Intracerebral Hemorrhage

Intracerebral hemorrhage (ICH), also known as cerebral bleed, is a type of intracranial bleed that occurs within the brain tissue or ventricles. Symptoms can include headache, one-sided weakness, vomiting, seizures, decreased level of consciousness, and neck stiffness. Often symptoms get worse over time. Fever is also common. In many cases bleeding is present in both the brain tissue and the ventricles.

Causes include brain trauma, aneurysms, arteriovenous malformations, and brain tumors. The largest risk factors for spontaneous bleeding are high blood pressure and amyloidosis. Other risk factors include alcoholism, low cholesterol, blood thinners, and cocaine. Diagnosis is typically by CT scan. Other conditions that may present similarly include ischemic stroke.

Treatment should typically be carried out in an intensive care unit. Guidelines recommended decreasing the blood pressure to a systolic of less than 140 mmHg. Blood thinners should be reversed if possible and blood sugar kept in the normal range. Surgery to place a ventricular drain may be used to treat hydrocephalus but corticosteroids should not be used. Surgery to remove the blood is useful in certain cases.

Cerebral bleeding affects about 2.5 per 10,000 people each year. It occurs more often in males and older people. About 44% of those affected die within a month. A good outcome occurs in about 20% of those affected. Strokes were first divided into their two major types, bleeding and insufficient blood flow, in 1823.

Signs and Symptoms

Patients with intraparenchymal bleeds have symptoms that correspond to the functions controlled by the area of the brain that is damaged by the bleed. Other symptoms include those that indicate a rise in intracranial pressure caused by a large mass putting pressure on the brain. Intracerebral hemorrhages are often misdiagnosed as subarachnoid hemorrhages due to the similarity in symptoms and signs. A severe headache followed by vomiting is one of the more common symptoms of intracerebral hemorrhage. Another common symptom is a patient can collapse. Some people may experience continuous bleeding from the ear. Some patients may also go into a coma before the bleed is noticed.

Causes

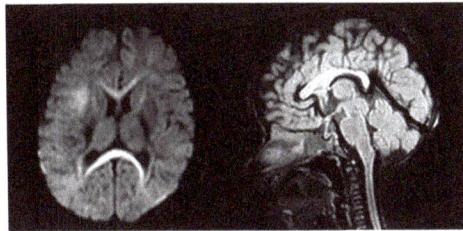

Splenial Infarct / Boomerang Sign, Sturge Weber Syndrome / Vein of Galen Malformation

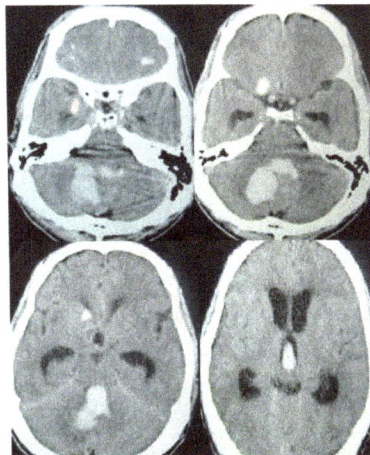

Axial CT scan showing hemorrhage in the posterior fossa

Intracerebral bleeds are the second most common cause of stroke, accounting for 10% of hospital admissions for stroke. High blood pressure raises the risks of spontaneous intracerebral hemorrhage by two to six times. More common in adults than in children, intraparenchymal bleeds are usually due to penetrating head trauma, but can also be due to depressed skull fractures. Acceleration-deceleration trauma, rupture of an aneurysm or arteriovenous malformation (AVM), and bleeding within a tumor are additional causes. Amyloid angiopathy is a not uncommon cause of intracerebral hemorrhage in patients over the age of 55. A very small proportion is due to cerebral venous sinus thrombosis.

Risk factors for ICH include:

- Hypertension (high blood pressure)

- Diabetes mellitus

- Menopause

- Cigarette smoking

- Excessive alcohol consumption

- Severe migraine

Tramautic intracerebral hematomas are divided into acute and delayed. Acute intracerebral hematomas occur at the time of the injury while delayed intracerebral hematomas have been reported from as early as 6 hours post injury to as long as several weeks.

Infection with the *k* serotype of *Streptococcus mutans* may also be a risk factor, because of its is more common in people who have had a stroke and productes collagen-binding protein.

Diagnosis

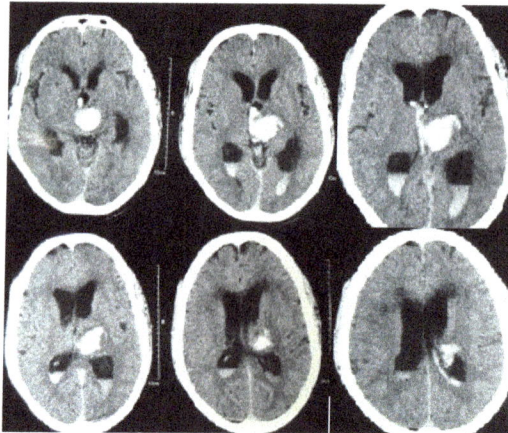

Spontaneous ICH with hydrocephalus on CT scan

Both computed tomography angiography (CTA) and magnetic resonance angiography (MRA) have been proved to be effective in diagnosing intracranial vascular malformations after ICH. So frequently, a CT angiogram will be performed in order to exclude a secondary cause of hemorrhage or to detect a "spot sign".

Intraparenchymal hemorrhage can be recognized on CT scans because blood appears brighter than other tissue and is separated from the inner table of the skull by brain tissue. The tissue surrounding a bleed is often less dense than the rest of the brain because of edema, and therefore shows up darker on the CT scan.

Location

When due to high blood pressure, they typically occur in the putamen or thalamus (60%), cerebrum (20%), cerebellum (13) or pons (7%).

Treatment

Treatment depends substantially of the type of ICH. Rapid CT scan and other diagnostic measures are used to determine proper treatment, which may include both medication and surgery.

- Tracheal intubation is indicated in people with decreased level of consciousness or other risk of airway obstruction.

- IV fluids are given to maintain fluid balance, using isotonic rather than hypotonic fluids.

Medication

- One review found that antihypertensive therapy to bring down the blood pressure in acute phases appears to improve outcomes. Other reviews found an unclear difference between intensive and less intensive blood pressure control. The American Heart Association and American Stroke Association guidelines in 2015 recommended decreasing the blood pressure to a SBP of 140 mmHg.

- Giving Factor VIIa within 4 hours limits the bleeding and formation of a hematoma. However, it also increases the risk of thromboembolism. It thus overall does not result in better outcomes in those without hemophilia.

- Frozen plasma, vitamin K, protamine, or platelet transfusions are given in case of a coagulopathy.

- Fosphenytoin or other anticonvulsant is given in case of seizures or lobar hemorrhage.

- H2 antagonists or proton pump inhibitors are commonly given for to try to prevent stress ulcers, a condition linked with ICH.

- Corticosteroids, were thought to reduce swelling. However, in large controlled studies, corticosteroids have been found to increase mortality rates and are no longer recommended.

Surgery

Surgery is required if the hematoma is greater than 3 cm (1 in), if there is a structural vascular lesion or lobar hemorrhage in a young patient.

- A catheter may be passed into the brain vasculature to close off or dilate blood vessels, avoiding invasive surgical procedures.

- Aspiration by stereotactic surgery or endoscopic drainage may be used in basal ganglia hemorrhages, although successful reports are limited.

Prognosis

The risk of death from an intraparenchymal bleed in traumatic brain injury is especially high when the injury occurs in the brain stem. Intraparenchymal bleeds within the medulla oblongata are almost always fatal, because they cause damage to cranial nerve X, the vagus nerve, which plays an important role in blood circulation and breathing. This kind of hemorrhage can also occur in the cortex or subcortical areas, usually in the frontal or temporal lobes when due to head injury, and sometimes in the cerebellum.

For spontaneous ICH seen on CT scan, the death rate (mortality) is 34–50% by 30 days after the insult, and half of the deaths occur in the first 2 days. Even though the majority of deaths occurs in the first days after ICH, survivors have a long term excess mortality of 27% compared to the general population.

The inflammatory response triggered by stroke has been viewed as harmful in the early stage, focusing on blood-borne leukocytes, neutrophils and macrophages, and resident microglia and astrocytes. A human postmortem study shows that inflammation occurs early and persists for several days after ICH. New area of interest are the Mast Cells.

Epidemiology

It accounts for 20% of all cases of cerebrovascular disease in the United States, behind cerebral thrombosis (40%) and cerebral embolism (30%).

It is two or more times more common in black than white people.

Wilderness Medical Emergency

A wilderness medical emergency is a medical emergency that takes place in a wilderness or remote setting at least 60 minutes away from definitive care (hospital, clinic, etc.). Such an emergency can require specialized skills, treatment techniques, and knowledge in order to manage the patient for an extended period of time before and during evacuation.

Types of Wilderness Medical Emergencies

Injury and Illness

- Arthropod bites and stings

- Appendicitis (leading to peritonitis folkloric "what if" for long distance sailing)

- Ballistic trauma (gunshot wound when hunting)

- Eye injuries (such as from branches)

- Flail chest associated with ice climbing and snowclimbing falls

- Hyperthermia (heat stroke or sunstroke)

    o Malignant hyperthermia

- Hypothermia

- Frostbite

- Poisoning

    o Food poisoning associated with warm weather expeditions

    o Venomous animal bite

    o Botanical from mushrooms or "wild greens""

- Severe burn (forest fire)

- Spreading wound infection

- Suspected spinal injury from falls, falling rock, ice

- Traumatic brain injury from falls, falling rock, ice

Infections Specific to Wilderness

- Lyme disease infection

- Malaria infection associated with expeditions

- Necrotizing Fasciitis

- Rabies infection

- Salmonella poisoning associated with expeditions

Neurological and Neurosurgical

- Subdural hematoma, associated with rockfall, icefall, falls while climbing, glissade crashes with rocks, mountain bike crashes

Respiratory

- Altitude sickness

- Asphyxia

- Drowning

- Smoke inhalation (related to Forest fire)

- Pneumothorax

- Pulmonary edema associated with high altitude (HAPE)

- Respiratory Arrest associated with neurotoxic bites

Shock

- Anaphylaxis associated with stings

- Hypovolemic shock (due to hemorrhage) associated with climbing falls, kayak crashes, etc.

- Septic shock

Mass-casualty Incidents

A mass casualty incident or MCI is an incident in which the number or severity of casualties overwhelms the available medical resources and service providers. Wilderness mass casualty incidents may include blizzards, earthquakes, avalanches, landslides, floods and forest fire, but they need not be natural disasters. Mass casualties have also been caused by human error in parties of climbers or explorers, with or without complications from inclement weather. In mass casualty incidents, emergency service providers must prioritize their patients using a process called triage in order to make the most of their limited resources.

Response

Extrication and Evacuation

Transporting an injured person out of the wilderness on a stretcher can be a difficult exercise requiring considerable manpower. It is advised that at least one person stay with an injured party and that no one attempt to seek help by travelling alone over inhospitable terrain.

Golden Hour

In emergency medicine, some advocates assert that there is a golden hour which refers to a time period lasting from a few minutes to several hours following traumatic injury being sustained by a casualty, during which there is the highest likelihood that prompt medical treatment will prevent death. While most medical professionals agree that delays in definitive care are undesirable, recent peer reviewed literature casts doubt on the validity of the 'golden hour' as it appears to lack a scientific basis. Dr. Bryan Bledsoe, an outspoken critic of the *golden hour* and other EMS "myths" like critical incident stress management, has indicated that the peer reviewed medical literature does not demonstrate any "magical time" for saving critical patients.

Responder Certifications

First Aid

Wilderness first aid (WFA) is the specific discipline of first aid which relates to care in remote areas, where emergency medical services will be difficult to obtain or will take a long time to arrive.

Locating the victim precedes assessment and intervention and in the case of wilderness response is often a difficult matter. Specialists in white water rescue, mountain rescue, mine disaster response and other fields are often employed. In some cases, emergency extrication procedures at incidents such as automobile accidents are required before assessment is possible. Only once the location of the victim has been determined, a trained responder has been dispatched and successfully reached the victim, can the ordinary first aid process begin. Assessment is then enabled and it follows carefully specified protocols which have been refined through a long process of evaluation.

Certification

Wilderness First Aid is a relatively new field compared to regular or 'urban' first aid. For this reason, there are a number of boards and societies which have been formed in recent years to attempt to establish normalized standards for wilderness first aid certification and wilderness medicine in general. Currently, there are no national standards for wilderness medicine, however one of the most popularly followed curricula is the

"National Practice Guidelines for Wilderness Emergency Care" published by the Wilderness Medical Society in 2010.

The American Red Cross Wilderness & Remote First Aid (r.2010) certification is valid for 2 years.

In Canada the first WFA courses were taught in the mid 1980s and the first organization to adopt standards was the Wilderness First Aid and Safety Association of BC (defunct since 1998).

As of 2014, all official BSA high adventure programs (such as Philmont) will require that at least two people (either an adviser or a youth participant) in each crew be currently certified in Wilderness First Aid or the equivalent and Adult CPR/AED from the American Red Cross, American Heart Association, Emergency Care and Safety Institute (ECSI), or American Safety & Health Institute (ASHI). At least one person must be certified in both WFA and CPR for all backpacking and camping activities where a Tour Plan must be filed. The preferred course is the American Red Cross Wilderness and Remote First Aid, which is a sixteen-hour course designed to help in situations where help is not readily available. Several hours may be required for high adventure staff to reach a remote backcountry location after a message is delivered to the nearest staffed camp. First aid and CPR training will result in proper and prompt attention being given to injuries and illnesses. Participants must present current certification cards upon check in to verify this requirement.

First Responders

A Wilderness First Responder (72- to 80-hour course) certification is both a higher certification than a Wilderness First Aid or (16- to 20-hour course) certification, and may also be used to upgrade an Emergency Medical Technician to a Wilderness Emergency Medical Technician. Outdoor Emergency Care is a National Ski Patrol certification, but it doesn't fully meet the requirements for a WFR certification.

Training and Certification Organizations

A number of fellowships are available for emergency medicine graduates including pre-hospital medicine (emergency medical services), hospice and palliative care, research, undersea and hyperbaric medicine, sports medicine, ultrasound, pediatric emergency medicine, disaster medicine, wilderness medicine, toxicology, and Critical Care Medicine.

- Wilderness Medicine Institute (WMI) of NOLS

- Wilderness Medicine Outfitters (WMO)

- Stonehearth Open Learning Opportunities (SOLO)

- True North Wilderness Survival School

- The Center for Wilderness Safety (CWS)

- American Red Cross

- American Safety & Health Institute (ASHI)

- Longleaf Wilderness Medicine (LWM)

- Survival Training School of California

References

- Whisnant JP (1996). "Effectiveness versus efficacy of treatment of hypertension for stroke prevention". Neurology. 46 (2): 301–7. doi:10.1212/WNL.46.2.301. PMID 8614485

- Small, Gary W (2002-06-22). "What we need to know about age related memory loss". British Medical Journal. 324 (7352): 1502–1507. doi:10.1136/bmj.324.7352.1502. PMC 1123445. PMID 12077041. Retrieved 2008-11-13

- McCaffrey RJ (1997). "Special Issues in the Evaluation of Mild Traumatic Brain Injury". The Practice of Forensic Neuropsychology: Meeting Challenges in the Courtroom. New York: Plenum Press. pp. 71–75. ISBN 0-306-45256-1

- NINDS (October 29, 2010). "Coma Information Page: National Institute of Neurological Disorders and Stroke (NINDS)". Retrieved 2010-12-08

- Hamilton M, Mrazik M, Johnson DW (July 2010). "Incidence of delayed intracranial hemorrhage in children after uncomplicated minor head injuries". Pediatrics. 126 (1): e33–9. doi:10.1542/peds.2009-0692. PMID 20566618

- Spodick, DH (Aug 14, 2003). "Acute cardiac tamponade.". The New England Journal of Medicine. 349 (7): 684–90. doi:10.1056/NEJMra022643. PMID 12917306

- Macfarlane, Robert; Hardy, David G. (1997). Outcome after Head, Neck and Spinal Trauma: a medicolegal guide. Oxford: Reed Educational and Professional Publishing Ltd. ISBN 0 7506 2178 8

- Eelco F.M. Wijdicks, MD; Coen A. Wijdicks, BS (2006). "The portrayal of coma in contemporary motion pictures". Neurology. 66 (9): 1300–1303. doi:10.1212/01.wnl.0000210497.62202.e9. PMID 16682658. Retrieved 2009-11-25

- Schiavone, WA (February 2013). "Cardiac tamponade: 12 pearls in diagnosis and management.". Cleveland Clinic journal of medicine. 80 (2): 109–16. doi:10.3949/ccjm.80a.12052. PMID 23376916

- Carlson, Neil R. (2013). "Physiology of Behavior". In Campanella, Craig. Neurological Disorders. Pearson Education, Inc. pp. 526–527. ISBN 0-205-23939-0

- "Pediatric Trauma And Triage: Overview of the Problem and Necessary Care for Positive Outcomes" (powerpoint). Jim Morehead. Retrieved 2010-11-06

- Debas, H. T.; Donkor, P.; Gawande, A.; Jamison, D. T.; Kruk, M. E.; Mock, C. N., eds. (2015). Essential Surgery. Disease Control Priorities. 1 (3rd ed.). Washington, DC: World Bank. doi:10.1596/978-1-4648-0346-8

- Stam J (April 2005). "Thrombosis of the cerebral veins and sinuses". The New England Journal of Medicine. 352 (17): 1791–8. doi:10.1056/NEJMra042354. PMID 15858188

- Seidenwurm DI (2007). "Introduction to brain imaging". In Brant WE, Helms CA. Fundamentals of Diagnostic Radiology. Philadelphia: Lippincott, Williams & Wilkins. p. 53. ISBN 0-7817-6135-2. Retrieved 2008-11-17

- Krug SE, Tuggle DW (2008). "Management of pediatric trauma" (PDF). Pediatrics. 121 (4): 849–54. doi:10.1542/peds.2008-0094. PMID 18381551. Retrieved 2010-11-06

- Guercini F, Acciarresi M, Agnelli G, Paciaroni M (April 2008). "Cryptogenic stroke: time to determine aetiology". Journal of Thrombosis and Haemostasis. 6 (4): 549–54. doi:10.1111/j.1538-7836.2008.02903.x. PMID 18208534

- Bordini, A.L.; Luiz, T.F.; Fernandes, M.; Arruda, W. O.; Teive, H. A. (2010). "Coma scales: a historical review". Arquivos de neuro-psiquiatria. 68 (6): 930–937. doi:10.1590/S0004-282X2010000600019. PMID 21243255

- Hannaman, Robert A. (2005). MedStudy Internal Medicine Review Core Curriculum: Neurology 11th Ed. MedStudy. pp. (11–1) to (11–2). ISBN 1-932703-01-2

- Hankey GJ (August 1999). "Smoking and risk of stroke". Journal of Cardiovascular Risk. 6 (4): 207–11. PMID 10501270

Emergency Medicine: An Integrated Study

The immediate medical attention given to patients suffering from illness and injury is known as emergency medicine. There are various models of emergency medicine across the world. The two commonly used models are specialist model and multidisciplinary model. This chapter has been carefully written to provide an easy understanding of the varied aspects of emergency medicine.

Emergency Medicine

Emergency medicine, formerly known in some countries as accident and emergency medicine, is the medical specialty involving care for undifferentiated and unscheduled patients with illnesses or injuries requiring immediate medical attention. In their role as first-line providers, emergency physicians are responsible for initiating investigations and interventions to diagnose and/or treat patients in the acute phase (including initial resuscitation and stabilization), coordinating care with physicians from other specialities, and making decisions regarding a patient's need for hospital admission, observation, or discharge. Emergency physicians generally practice in hospital emergency departments, pre-hospital settings via emergency medical services, and intensive care units, but may also work in primary care settings such as urgent care clinics.

Different models for emergency medicine exist internationally. In countries following the Anglo-American model, emergency medicine was originally the domain of surgeons, general practitioners, and other generalist physicians, but in recent decades it has become recognised as a speciality in its own right with its own training programmes and academic posts, and the specialty is now a popular choice among medical students and newly qualified medical practitioners. By contrast, in countries following the Franco-German model, the speciality does not exist and emergency medical care is instead provided directly by anesthesiologists (for initial resuscitation), surgeons, specialists in internal medicine, or another speciality as appropriate. In developing countries, emergency medicine is still evolving and international emergency medicine programs offer hope of improving basic emergency care where resources are limited.

Scope

Emergency Medicine is a medical specialty—a field of practice based on the knowledge and skills required for the prevention, diagnosis and management of acute and urgent aspects of illness and injury affecting patients of all age groups with a full spectrum of undifferentiated physical and behavioral disorders. It further encompasses an understanding of the development of pre-hospital and in-hospital emergency medical systems and the skills necessary for this development.

The field of emergency medicine encompasses care involving the acute care of internal medical and surgical conditions. In many modern emergency departments, Emergency physicians are tasked with seeing a large number of patients, treating their illnesses and arranging for disposition—either admitting them to the hospital or releasing them after treatment as necessary. The emergency physician requires a broad field of knowledge and advanced procedural skills often including surgical procedures, trauma resuscitation, advanced cardiac life support and advanced airway management. They must have the skills of many specialists—the ability to resuscitate a patient (critical care medicine), manage a difficult airway (anesthesia), suture a complex laceration (plastic surgery), reduce (set) a fractured bone or dislocated joint (orthopedic surgery), treat a heart attack (cardiology), manage strokes (neurology), work-up a pregnant patient with vaginal bleeding (obstetrics and gynecology), stop a severe nosebleed (ENT), place a chest tube (cardiothoracic surgery), and to conduct and interpret x-rays and ultrasounds (radiology). Emergency physicians also provide episodic primary care to patients during off hours and for those who do not have primary care providers.

Emergency medicine is distinct from urgent care, which refers to immediate healthcare for less emergent medical issues. However, many emergency physicians work in urgent care settings, since there is obvious overlap. Emergency medicine also includes many aspects of acute primary care, and shares with family medicine the uniqueness of seeing all patients regardless of age, gender or organ system . The emergency physician workforce also includes many competent physicians who trained in other specialties.

Physicians specializing in emergency medicine can enter fellowships to receive credentials in subspecialties such as palliative care, critical-care medicine, medical toxicology, wilderness medicine, pediatric emergency medicine, sports medicine, disaster medicine, tactical medicine, ultrasound, pain medicine, pre-hospital emergency medicine, or undersea and hyperbaric medicine.

The practice of emergency medicine is often quite different in rural areas where there are far fewer consultants and health care resources. In these areas, family physicians with additional skills in emergency medicine often staff emergency departments. Rural emergency physicians may be the only health care providers in the community, and require skills that include primary care and obstetrics.

Work Patterns

Patterns vary by country and region. In the United States, the employment arrangement of emergency physician practices are either private (with a co-operative group of doctors staffing an emergency department under contract), institutional (physicians with an independent contractor relationship with the hospital), corporate (physicians with an independent contractor relationship with a third-party staffing company that services multiple emergency departments), or governmental (for example, when working within®personal service military services, public health services, veterans' benefit systems or other government agencies).

In the United Kingdom, all consultants in emergency medicine work in the National Health Service and there is little scope for private emergency practice. In other countries like Australia, New Zealand or Turkey, emergency medicine specialists are almost always salaried employees of government health departments and work in public hospitals, with pockets of employment in private or non-government aeromedical rescue or transport services, as well as some private hospitals with emergency departments; they may be supplemented or backed by non-specialist medical officers, and visiting general practitioners. Rural emergency departments may be headed by general practitioners alone, sometimes with non-specialist qualifications in emergency medicine.

History

During the French Revolution, after seeing the speed with which the carriages of the French flying artillery maneuvered across the battlefields, French military surgeon Dominique Jean Larrey applied the idea of ambulances, or "flying carriages", for rapid transport of wounded soldiers to a central place where medical care was more accessible and effective. Larrey manned ambulances with trained crews of drivers, corpsmen and litter-bearers and had them bring the wounded to centralized field hospitals, effectively creating a forerunner of the modern MASH units. Dominique Jean Larrey is sometimes called the father of emergency medicine for his strategies during the French wars.

Emergency medicine as an independent medical specialty is relatively young. Prior to the 1960s and 1970s, hospital emergency departments (EDs) were generally staffed by physicians on staff at the hospital on a rotating basis, among them family physicians, general surgeons, internists, and a variety of other specialists. In many smaller emergency departments, nurses would triage patients and physicians would be called in based on the type of injury or illness. Family physicians were often on call for the emergency department, and recognized the need for dedicated emergency department coverage. Many of the pioneers of emergency medicine were family physicians and other specialists who saw a need for additional training in emergency care.

During this period, groups of physicians began to emerge who had left their respective practices in order to devote their work completely to the ED. In the UK in 1952, Maurice Ellis was appointed as the first "casualty consultant" at Leeds General Infirmary. In 1967, the Casualty Surgeons Association was established with Maurice Ellis as its first President. In the US, the first of such groups was headed by Dr. James DeWitt Mills in 1961 who, along with four associate physicians; Dr. Chalmers A. Loughridge, Dr. William Weaver, Dr. John McDade, and Dr. Steven Bednar at Alexandria Hospital, Virginia, established 24/7 year-round emergency care, which became known as the "Alexandria Plan".

It was not until the establishment of American College of Emergency Physicians (ACEP), the recognition of emergency medicine training programs by the AMA and the AOA, and in 1979 a historical vote by the American Board of Medical Specialties that emergency medicine became a recognized medical specialty in the US. The first emergency medicine residency program in the world was begun in 1970 at the University of Cincinnati and the first Department of Emergency Medicine at a US medical school was founded in 1971 at the University of Southern California.

In 1990 the UK's Casualty Surgeons Association changed its name to the British Association for Accident and Emergency Medicine, and subsequently became the British Association for Emergency Medicine (BAEM) in 2004. In 1993, an intercollegiate Faculty of Accident and Emergency Medicine (FAEM) was formed as a "daughter college" of six medical royal colleges in England and Scotland to arrange professional examinations and training. In 2005, the BAEM and the FAEM were merged to form the College of Emergency Medicine, now the Royal College of Emergency Medicine, which conducts membership and fellowship examinations and publishes guidelines and standards for the practise of emergency medicine.

Financing and Practice Organization

Reimbursement

Many hospitals and care centers feature departments of emergency medicine, where patients can receive acute care without an appointment. While many patients are treated for life-threatening injuries, others utilize the emergency department (ED) for non-urgent reasons such as headaches or a cold. (defined as "visits for conditions for which a delay of several hours would not increase the likelihood of an adverse outcome"). As such, EDs can adjust staffing ratios and designate an area of the department for faster patient turnover to accommodate a variety of patient needs and volumes. Policies have been developed to better assist ED staff(such as Emergency Medical Technicians, paramedics, and mid level providers such as nurses and physicians assistants) direct patients towards more appropriate medical settings, such as their primary care physician, urgent care clinics or detoxification facilities. The emergency department, along with welfare programs and healthcare clinics, serves as a critical part of the healthcare safety net for patients who are uninsured, cannot afford medical treatment or do not understand how to properly utilize their coverage.

Compensation

Emergency physicians are compensated at a higher rate in comparison to some other specialities, ranking 10th out of 26 physician specialties in 2015, at an average salary of $306,000 annually. They are compensated in the mid-range (averaging $13,000 annually) for non-patient activities, such as speaking engagements or acting as an expert witness; they also saw a 12% increase in salary from 2014 - 2015 (which was not out of line with many other physician specialties that year). While emergency physicians work 8-12 hour shifts and do not tend to work on-call, the high level of stress and need for strong diagnostic and triage capabilities for the undifferentiated, acute patient contributes to arguments justifying higher salaries for these physicians. Emergency care must be available every hour of every day, and requires a doctor to be available on site 24/7, unlike an outpatient clinic or some other hospital departments that have more limited hours, and may only call a physician in when needed. The necessity to have a physician on staff along with all other diagnostic services available every hour of every day is thus a costly arrangement for hospitals.

Payment Systems

American health payment systems are undergoing significant reform efforts, which include compensating emergency physicians through "Pay for Performance" incentives and penalty measures under commercial and public health programs, including Medicare and Medicaid. This payment reform aims to improve quality of care and control costs, despite the differing opinions on the existing evidence to show that this payment approach is effective in emergency medicine. Initially, these incentives were only targeted toward primary care providers (PCPs), but some would argue emergency medicine is primary care, as no one refers patients to the ED. In one such program, two specific conditions listed were directly tied to patients frequently seen by emergency medical providers: acute myocardial infarction and pneumonia.

There are some challenges with implementing these quality-based incentives in emergency medicine in that patients are often not given a definitive diagnosis in the ED, making it difficult to allocate payments through coding. Additionally, adjustments based on patient risk-level and multiple co-morbidities for complex patients further complicate attribution of positive or negative health outcomes, and it is difficult to assess whether much of the costs are a direct result of the emergent condition being treated in acute care settings. It is also difficult to quantify the savings due to preventive care during emergency treatment (i.e. workup, stabilizing treatments, coordination of care and discharge, rather than a hospital admission). Thus, ED providers tend to support a modified fee-for-service model over other payment systems.

Overutilization

Some patients without health insurance utilize EDs as their primary form of medical care. Because these patients do not utilize insurance or primary care, emergency medical providers often face problems of overutilization and financial loss, especially since many patients are unable to pay for their care. ED overuse produces $38 billion in wasteful spending each year (i.e. care delivery and coordination failures, over-treat-ment, administrative complexity, pricing failures, and fraud), and unnecessarily drains departmental resources, reducing the quality of care across all patients. While over-use is not limited to the uninsured, the uninsured comprise a growing proportion of non-urgent ED visits – insurance coverage can help mitigate overutilization by im-proving access to alternative forms of care and lowering the need for emergency vis-its. A common misconception pegs frequent ED visitors as a major factor in wasteful spending. However, frequent ED users make up a small portion of those contributing to overutilization and are often insured.

Uncompensated Care

Injury and illness are often unforeseen, and patients of lower socioeconomic status are especially susceptible to being suddenly burdened with the cost of a necessary ED visit. If they are unable to pay for the care they received, then the hospital (which under the Emergency Medical Treatment and Active Labor Act (EMTALA), as discussed below, is obligated to treat emergency conditions regardless of ability to pay) faces an economic loss for this uncompensated care. Fifty-five percent of emergency care is uncompensat-ed, and inadequate reimbursement has led to the closure of many EDs. Policy changes (such as the Affordable Care Act) designed to decrease the number of uninsured people have been projected to drastically lower the amount of uncompensated care.

In addition to decreasing the uninsured rate, ED overutilization might be mitigated by improving patient access to primary care and increasing patient flow to alternative care centers for non-life threatening injuries. Financial disincentives, patient education, as well as improved management for patients with chronic diseases can also reduce over-utilization and help to manage costs of care. Moreover, physician knowledge of prices for treatment and analyses, discussions on costs with their patients, as well as a chang-ing culture away from defensive medicine can improve cost-effective use. A transition towards more value-based care in the ED is an avenue by which providers can contain costs.

EMTALA

Doctors that work in the EDs of hospitals receiving Medicare funding are subject to the provisions of EMTALA. EMTALA was enacted by the US Congress in 1986 to cur-tail "patient dumping," a practice whereby patients were refused medical care for eco-nomic or other non-medical reasons. Since its enactment, ED visits have substantially increased, with one study showing a rise in visits of 26% (which is more than double the increase in population over the same period of time). While more individuals are receiving care, a lack of funding and ED overcrowding may be impacting quality. To comply with the provisions of EMTALA, hospitals, through their ED physicians, must provide a medical screening and stabilize the emergency medical conditions of anyone that presents themselves at a hospital ED with patient capacity. If these services are not provided, EMTALA holds both the hospital and the responsible ED physician liable for civil penalties of up to $50,000 each. While both the Office of Inspector General, U.S. Department of Health and Human Services (OIG) and private citizens can bring an action under EMTALA, courts have uniformly held that ED physicians can only be held liable if the case is prosecuted by OIG (whereas hospitals are subject to penalties regardless of who brings the suit). Additionally, the Center for Medicare and Medicaid Services (CMS) can discontinue provider status under Medicare for physicians that do not comply with EMTALA. Liability also extends to on-call physicians that fail to respond to an ED request to come to the hospital to provide service. While the goals of EMTALA are laudable, commentators have noted that it appears to have created a substantial unfunded burden on the resources of hospitals and emergency physicians. As a result of financial difficulty, between the period of 1991-2011, 12.6% of EDs in the US closed.

Care Delivery in Different ED Settings

Rural

Despite the practice emerging over the past few decades, the delivery of emergency medicine has significantly increased and evolved across diverse settings as it relates to cost, provider availability and overall usage. Prior to the Affordable Care Act (ACA), emergency medicine was leveraged primarily by "uninsured or underinsured patients, women, children, and minorities, all of whom frequently face barriers to accessing primary care". While this still exists today to an extent as mentioned above, it is critical to consider the location in which care is delivered to understand the population and system challenges related to overutilization and high cost. In rural communities where provider and ambulatory facility shortages exist, a primary care physician (PCP) in the ED with general knowledge is likely to be the only source of health care for a population, as specialists and other health resources are generally unavailable due to lack of funding and desire to serve in these areas. Unfortunately as a result, the incidence of complex co-morbidities not managed by the appropriate provider results in worse health outcomes and eventually costlier care that extends beyond rural communities. Though typically quite separated, it is crucial that PCPs in rural areas partner with larger health systems to comprehensively address the complex needs of their community, improve population health, and implement strategies such as telemedicine to positively impact health outcomes and reduce ED utilization for preventative illnesses.

Urban

Alternatively, emergency medicine in urban areas consists of diverse provider groups including PCPs, nurse practitioners, physicians, and registered nurses who coordinate with specialists in both inpatient and outpatient facilities to address patients' needs, more specifically in the ED. For all systems regardless of funding source, EMTALA mandates EDs to conduct a medical examination for anyone that presents at the department, irrespective of paying ability. Fortunately, non-profit hospitals and health systems - as required by the ACA - must provide a certain threshold of charity care "by actively ensuring that those who qualify for financial assistance get it, by charging reasonable rates to uninsured patients and by avoiding extraordinary collection practices". While there are limitations, this mandate provides support to many in need. That said, despite policy efforts and increased funding and federal reimbursement in urban areas, the triple aim (of improving patient experience, enhancing population health, and reducing the per-capita cost of care) remains a challenge without providers' and payers' collaboration to increase access to preventive care and decrease in ED usage. As a result, many experts support the notion that emergency medical services should serve only immediate risks in both urban and rural areas.

Patient-Provider Relationships

As stated above, EMTALA includes provisions that protect patients from being turned away or transferred before adequate stabilization. Upon making contact with a patient, EMS providers have a responsibility to diagnose and stabilize a patient's condition without regard for ability to pay. In the prehospital setting, providers must exercise appropriate judgement in choosing a suitable hospital for transport. Hospitals can only turn away incoming ambulances if they are on diversion and incapable of providing adequate care. However, once a patient has arrived on hospital property, care must be provided. At the hospital, contact with the patient is first made by a triage nurse who determines the appropriate level of care needed.

According to the Mead v. Legacy Health System, a patient-physician relationship is established when "the physician takes an affirmative action with regard to the care of the patient". Initiating such a relationship forms a legal contract in which the physician must continue to provide treatment or properly terminate the relationship. This legal responsibility can extend to physician consultations and on-call physicians even without direct patient contact. In emergency medicine, termination of the patient-provider relationship prior to stabilization or without handoff to another qualified provider is considered abandonment. In order to initiate an outside transfer, a physician must verify that the next hospital can provide a similar or higher level of care. Hospitals and physicians must also ensure that the patient's condition will not be further aggravated by the transfer process.

The unique setting of emergency medicine practice presents a challenge for delivering high quality, patient-centered care. Clear, effective communication can be particularly difficult due to noise, frequent interruptions, and high patient turnover. The Society for Academic Emergency Medicine has identified five tasks that are essential to patient-physician communication: establishing rapport, gathering information, giving information, providing comfort, and collaboration. The miscommunication of patient information is a key source of medical error; minimizing shortcoming in communication remains a topic of current and future research.

Medical Error

Many circumstances, including the regular transfer of patients in the course of emergency treatment, and crowded, noisy and chaotic ED environments, make emergency medicine particularly susceptible to medical error and near misses. One study identified an error rate of 18 per 100 registered patients in one particular academic ED. Another study found that where a lack of teamwork (i.e. poor communication, lack of team structure, lack of cross-monitoring) was implicated in a particular incident of ED medical error, "an average of 8.8 teamwork failures occurred per case [and] more than half of the deaths and permanent disabilities that occurred were judged avoidable." Unfortunately, certain cultural (i.e. "a focus on the errors of others and a 'blame-and-shame' culture") and structural (i.e. lack of standardization and equipment incompatibilities) aspects of emergency medicine often result in a lack of disclosure of medical error and near misses to patients and other caregivers. While concerns about malpractice liability is one reason why disclosure of medical errors is not made, some have noted that disclosing the error and providing an apology can mitigate malpractice risk. Ethicists uniformly agree that the disclosure of a medical error that causes harm is the duty of a care provider. The key components of disclosure include "honesty, explanation, empathy, apology, and the chance to lessen the chance of future errors" (represented by the mnemonic HEEAL). The nature of emergency medicine is such that error will likely always be a substantial risk of emergency care. Maintaining public trust through open communication regarding harmful error, however, can help patients and physicians constructively address problems when they occur.

Treatments

Emergency Medicine is a primary, or first-contact point of care for patients requiring the use of the health care system. Specialists in Emergency Medicine are required to possess specialist skills in acute illness diagnosis and resuscitation. Emergency physician are responsible for providing immediate recognition, evaluation, care, stabilization, to \adult and pediatric patients in response to acute illness and injury.

Training

There are a variety of international models for emergency medicine training. Among those with well developed training programs there are two different models: a "specialist" model or "a multidisciplinary model". Additionally, in some countries the emergency medicine specialist rides in the ambulance. For example, in France and Germany the physician, often an anesthesiologist, rides in the ambulance and provides stabilizing care at the scene. The patient is then triaged to the appropriate department of a hospital, so emergency care is much more multidisciplinary than in the Anglo-American model.

In countries such as the US, the United Kingdom, Canada and Australia, ambulances crewed by paramedics and emergency medical technicians respond to out-of-hospital emergencies and transport patients to emergency departments, meaning there is more dependence on these health-care providers and there is more dependence on paramedics and EMTs for on-scene care. Emergency physicians are therefore more "specialists", since all patients are taken to the emergency department. Most developing countries follow the Anglo-American model: 3 or 4 year independent residency training programs in emergency medicine are the gold standard. Some countries develop training programs based on a primary care foundation with additional emergency medicine training. In developing countries, there is an awareness that Western models may not be applicable and may not be the best use of limited health care resources. For example, specialty training and pre-hospital care like that in developed countries is too expensive and impractical for use in many developing countries with limited health care resources. International emergency medicine provides an important global perspective and hope for improvement in these areas.

A brief review of some of these programs follows:

Argentina

In Argentina, the SAE (Sociedad Argentina de Emergencias) is the main organization of Emergency Medicine. There are a lot of residency programs. Also it is possible to reach the certification with a two-year postgraduate university course after a few years of ED background.

Australia and New Zealand

The specialist medical college responsible for Emergency Medicine in Australia and New Zealand is the Australasian College for Emergency Medicine (ACEM). The training program is nominally seven years in duration, after which the trainee is awarded a Fellowship of ACEM, conditional upon passing all necessary assessments.

Dual fellowship programs also exist for Paediatric Medicine (in conjunction with the Royal Australasian College of Physicians) and Intensive Care Medicine (in conjunction with the College of Intensive Care Medicine). These programs nominally add one or more years to the ACEM training program.

For medical doctors not (and not wishing to be) specialists in Emergency Medicine but have a significant interest or workload in emergency departments, the ACEM provides non-specialist certificates and diplomas.

Canada

The two routes to emergency medicine certification can be summarized as follows:

1. A 5-year residency leading to the designation of FRCP(EM) through the Royal

College of Physicians and Surgeons of Canada (Emergency Medicine Board Certification - Emergency Medicine Consultant).

2. A 1-year emergency medicine enhanced skills program following a 2-year family medicine residency leading to the designation of CCFP(EM) through the College of Family Physicians of Canada (Advanced Competency Certification). The CFPC also allows those having worked a minimum of 4 years at a minimum of 400 hours per year in emergency medicine to challenge the examination of special competence in emergency medicine and thus become specialized.

CCFP(EM) emergency physicians outnumber FRCP(EM) physicians by a ratio of about 3 to 1, and they tend to work primarily as clinicians with a smaller focus on academic activities such as teaching and research. FRCP(EM) Emergency Medicine Board specialists tend to congregate in academic centers and tend to have more academically oriented careers, which emphasize administration, research, critical care, disaster medicine, and teaching. They also tend to sub-specialize in toxicology, critical care, pediatrics emergency medicine, and sports medicine. Furthermore, the length of the FRCP(EM) residency allows more time for formal training in these areas.

China

The current post-graduate Emergency Medicine training process is highly complex in China. The first EM post-graduate training took place in 1984 at the Peking Union Medical College Hospital. Because specialty certification in EM has not been established, formal training is not required to practice Emergency Medicine in China.

About a decade ago, Emergency Medicine residency training was centralized at the municipal levels, following the guidelines issued by The Ministry of Public Health. Residency programs in all hospitals are called residency training bases, which have to be approved by local health governments. These bases are hospital-based, but the residents are selected and managed by the municipal associations of medical education. These associations are also the authoritative body of setting up their residents' training curriculum. All medical school graduates wanting to practice medicine have to go through 5 years of residency training at designated training bases, first 3 years of general rotation followed by 2 more years of specialty-centered training.

Germany

In Germany, emergency medicine is not handled as a specialisation (Facharztrichtung), but any licensed physician can acquire an additional qualification in emergency medicine through an 80-hour course monitored by the respective *"Ärztekammer"* (medical association, responsible for licensing of physicians). A service as emergency physician in an ambulance service is part of the specialisation training of anaesthesiology. Emergency physicians usually work on a volunteering basis and are often anaesthesiologists, but may be specialists of any kind.

India

India is an example of how family medicine can be a foundation for emergency medicine training. Many private hospitals and institutes have been providing Emergency Medicine training for doctors, nurses & paramedics since 1994, with certification programs varying from 6 months to 3 years. However, emergency medicine was only recognized as a separate specialty by the Medical Council of India in July 2009.

Malaysia

There are three universities (Universiti Sains Malaysia, Universiti Kebangsaan Malaysia, & Universiti Malaya) that offer master's degrees in emergency medicine - postgraduate training programs of four years in duration with clinical rotations, examinations and a dissertation. The first cohort of locally trained emergency physicians graduated in 2002.

Saudi Arabia

In Saudi Arabia, Certification of Emergency Medicine is done by taking the 4-year program Saudi Board of Emergency Medicine (SBEM), which is accredited by Saudi Council for Health Specialties (SCFHS). It requires passing the two-part exam: first part and final part (written and oral) to obtain the SBEM certificate, which is equivalent to Doctorate Degree.

United States

Most programs are three years in duration, but some programs are four years long. There are several combined residencies offered with other programs including family medicine, internal medicine and pediatrics. The US is well known for its excellence in emergency medicine residency training programs. This has led to some controversy about specialty certification.

There are three ways to become board-certified in emergency medicine:

- The American Board of Emergency Medicine (ABEM) is for those with either Doctor of Medicine (MD) or Doctor of Osteopathic Medicine (DO) degrees. The ABEM is under the authority of the American Board of Medical Specialties.

- The American Osteopathic Board of Emergency Medicine (AOBEM) certifies only emergency physicians with a DO degree. It is under the authority of the American Osteopathic Association Bureau of Osteopathic Specialists.

- • The Board of Certification in Emergency Medicine (BCEM) grants board certification in emergency medicine to physicians who have not completed an emergency medicine residency, but have completed a residency in other fields (internists, family practitioners, pediatricians, general surgeons, and anesthesiologists).

A number of ABMS fellowships are available for Emergency Medicine graduates including pre-hospital medicine (emergency medical services), critical care, hospice and palliative care, research, undersea and hyperbaric medicine, sports medicine, pain medicine, ultrasound, pediatric Emergency Medicine, disaster medicine, wilderness medicine, toxicology, and critical care medicine.

In recent years, workforce data has led to a recognition of the need for additional training for primary care physicians who provide emergency care.

This has led to a number of supplemental training programs in first hour emergency care, and a few fellowships for family physicians in emergency medicine.

Funding for Training

"In 2010, there were 157 allopathic and 37 osteopathic emergency medicine residency programs, which collectively accept about 2,000 new residents each year. Studies have shown that attending emergency physician supervision of residents directly correlates to a higher quality and more cost-effective practice, especially when an emergency medicine residency exists." Medical education is primarily funded through the Medicare program; payments are given to hospitals for each resident. "Fifty-five percent of ED payments come from Medicare, fifteen percent from Medicaid, five percent from private payment and twenty-five percent from commercially insured patients." However, choices of physician specialties are not mandated by any agency or program, so even though emergency departments see many Medicare/Medicaid patients, and thus receive a lot of funding for training from these programs, there is still concern over a shortage of specialty-trained Emergency Medicine providers.

United Kingdom

In the United Kingdom, the Royal College of Emergency Medicine has a role in setting the professional standards and the assessment of trainees. Emergency medical trainees enter specialty training after five or six years of Medical school followed by two years of foundation training. Specialty training takes six years to complete and success in the assessments and a set of five examinations results in the award of Fellowship of the Royal College of Emergency Medicine (FRCEM).

Historically, emergency specialists were drawn from anaesthesia, medicine, and surgery. Many established EM consultants were surgically trained; some hold the Fellowship of Royal College of Surgeons of Edinburgh in Accident and Emergency — FRCSEd(A&E). Trainees in Emergency Medicine may dual accredit in Intensive care medicine or seek sub-specialisation in Paediatric Emergency Medicine.

Turkey

Emergency Medicine residency lasts for 4 years in Turkey. These physicians have a 2-year Obligatory Service in Turkey to be qualified to have their diploma. After this period, EM specialist can choose to work in private or governmental ED's.

Pakistan

Emergency Medicine training in Pakistan lasts for 5 years. The initial 2 years involve trainees to be sent to three major areas which include Medicine and allied, Surgery and Allied and critical care. It is divided into six months each and the rest six months out of first two years are spent in emergency department. In last three years trainee residents spend most of their time in emergency room as senior residents. Certificate courses include ACLS, PALS, ATLS, and research and dissertations are required for successful completion of the training. At the end of 5 years, candidates become eligible for sitting for FCPS part II exam. After fulfilling the requirement they become fellow of College of Physicians and Surgeons Pakistan in Emergency Medicine.

Presently there are two institutions where you can acquire this training which are Shifa International Hospitals Islamabad and Aga Khan Hospital Karachi. there are approximately 30 residents in different years of training, while the College has conducted its first exit examination for the FCPS in Emergency Medicine during December 2015.

Iran

The first residency program in Iran started in 2002 at Iran University of Medical Sciences, and there are now three-year standard residency programs running in Tehran, Tabriz, Mashhad, Isfahan, and some other universities. All these programs work under supervision of Emergency Medicine specialty board committee. There are now more than 200 (and increasing) board-certified Emergency Physicians in Iran.

Ethical and Medicolegal Issues

Ethical and medico-legal issues are embedded within the nature of Emergency Medicine. Issues surrounding competence, end of life care, and right to refuse care are encountered on a daily basis within the Emergency Department. Of growing significance are the ethical issues and legal obligations that surround the Mental Health Act, as increasing numbers of suicide attempts and self harm are seen in the Emergency Department The Wooltorton case of 2007 in which a patient arrived at the Emergency Department post overdose with a note specifying her request for no interventions, highlights the dichotomy that often exists between a physicians ethical obligation to 'do no harm' and the legality of a patients right to refuse.

Emergency Medical Technician

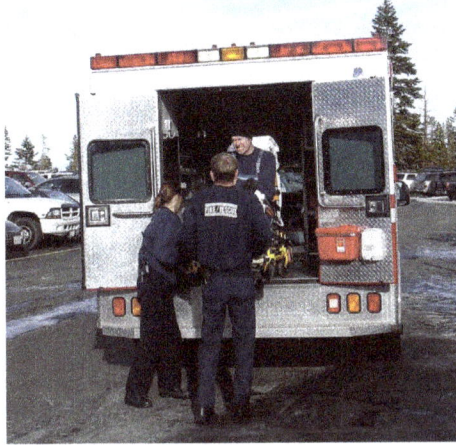

EMTs loading an injured skier into an ambulance.

Emergency Medical Technician (EMT) and ambulance technician are terms used in some countries to denote a health care provider of emergency medical services. EMTs are clinicians, trained to respond quickly to emergency situations regarding medical issues, traumatic injuries and accident scenes. Under the British system and those that are influenced by it, they are referred to as ambulance technicians (often shortened to techs), while in the American system and its influenced countries, they are referred to as emergency medical technicians.

EMTs are most commonly found working in ambulances, but should not be confused with "ambulance drivers" or "ambulance attendants" – ambulance staff who in the past were not trained in emergency care or driving. EMTs are often employed by private ambulance services, governments, and hospitals, but are also often employed by fire departments (and seen on fire apparatus), in police departments (and seen on police vehicles), and there are many firefighter/EMTs and police officer/EMTs. EMTs operate under a limited scope of practice. EMTs are normally supervised by a medical director, who is a physician.

Some EMTs are paid employees, while others (particularly those in rural areas) are volunteers.

Canada

There is considerable degree of inter-provincial variation in the Canadian Paramedic practice. Although a national consensus (by way of the National Occupational Competency Profile) identifies certain knowledge, skills, and abilities as being most synonymous with a given level of Paramedic practice, each province retains ultimate authority in legislating the actual administration and delivery of emergency medical services within its own borders. For this reason, any discussion of *Paramedic Practice* in Canada is necessarily broad, and general. Specific regulatory frameworks and questions related to Paramedic practice can only definitively be answered by consulting relevant provincial legislation, although provincial Paramedic Associations may often offer a simpler overview of this topic when it is restricted to a province-by-province basis.

In Canada, the levels of paramedic practice as defined by the National Occupational Competency Profile are: Emergency Medical Responder (EMR), Primary Care Paramedic, Advanced Care Paramedic, and Critical Care Paramedic.

Regulatory frameworks vary from province to province, and include direct government regulation (such as Ontario's method of credentialing its practitioners with the title of A-EMCA, or Advanced Emergency Medical Care Assistant) to professional self-regulating bodies, such as the Alberta College of Paramedics. Though the title of Paramedic is a generic description of a category of practitioners, provincial variability in regulatory methods accounts for ongoing differences in actual titles that are ascribed to different levels of practitioners. For example, the province of Alberta has legally adopted the title "Emergency Medical Technician", or 'EMT', for the Primary Care Paramedic; and 'Paramedic' only for those qualified as Advanced Care Paramedics Advanced Life Support (ALS) providers. Only someone registered in Alberta can call themselves an EMT or Paramedic in Alberta, the title is legally protected. Almost all other provinces are gradually moving to adopting the new titles, or have at least recognized the NOCP document as a benchmarking document to permit inter-provincial labour mobility of practitioners, regardless of how titles are specifically regulated within their own provincial systems. In this manner, the confusing myriad of titles and occupational descriptions can at least be discussed using a common language for comparison sake.

Emergency Medical Responder

Most providers that work in ambulances will be identified as 'Paramedics' by the public. However, in many cases, the most prevalent level of emergency prehospital care is that which is provided by the Emergency Medical Responder (EMR). This is a level of practice recognized under the National Occupational Competency Profile, although unlike the next three successive levels of practice, the EMR is not specifically considered a Paramedic, *per se*. The high number of EMRs across Canada cannot be ignored as contributing a critical role in the chain of survival, although it is a level of practice that is least comprehensive (clinically speaking), and is also generally not consistent with any medical acts beyond advanced first-aid and oxygen therapy, with the exception of automated external defibrillation (which is still considered a regulated medical act in most provinces in Canada).

Primary Care Paramedics

Primary care paramedics (PCP) are the entry-level of paramedic practice in Canadian provinces. The scope of practice includes performing semi-automated external defibrillation, interpretation of 4-lead ECGs, administration of Symptom Relief Medications for a variety of emergency medical conditions (these include oxygen, epinephrine, dextrose, glucagon, salbutamol, ASA and nitroglycerine), performing trauma immobilization (including cervical immobilization), and other fundamental basic medical care. Primary Care Paramedics may also receive additional training in order to perform certain skills that are normally in the scope of practice of Advanced Care Paramedics. This is regulated both provincially (by statute) and locally (by the medical director), and ordinarily entails an aspect of medical oversight by a specific body or group of physicians. This is often referred to as Medical Control, or a role played by a base hospital. For example, in the provinces of Ontario and Newfoundland and Labrador, many paramedic services allow Primary Care Paramedics to perform 12-lead ECG interpretation, or initiate intravenous therapy to deliver a few additional medications.

Advanced Care Paramedics

The Advanced Care Paramedic is a level of practitioner that is in high demand by many services across Canada. However, still not all provinces and jurisdictions have ACPs (Quebec, New Brunswick). The ACP typically carries approximately 20 different medications, although the number and type of medications may vary substantially from region to region. ACPs perform advanced airway management including intubation, surgical airways, intravenous therapy, place external jugular IV lines, perform needle thoracotomy, perform and interpret 12-lead ECGs, perform synchronized and chemical cardioversion, transcutaneous pacing, perform obstetrical assessments, and provide pharmacological pain relief for various conditions. Several sites in Canada have adopted pre-hospital fibrinolytics and rapid sequence induction, and prehospital medical research has permitted a great number of variations in the scope of practice for ACPs. Current programs include providing ACPs with discretionary direct 24-hour access to PCI labs, bypassing the emergency department, and representing a fundamental change in both the way that patients with S-T segment elevation myocardial infarctions (STEMI) are treated, but also profoundly affecting survival rates. as well as bypassing a closer hospitals to get an identified stroke patient to a stroke centre.

Critical Care Paramedic

Critical Care Paramedics (CCPs) are paramedics who generally do not respond to 9-1-1 emergency calls, with the exception of helicopter "scene" calls. Instead they focus on transferring patients from the hospital they are currently in to other hospitals that can provide a higher level of care. CCPs often work in collaboration with registered nurses and respiratory therapists during hospital transfers. This ensures continuity of care. However, when acuity is manageable by a CCP or a registered nurse or respiratory therapist is not available, CCPs will work alone. Providing this care to the patient allows the sending hospital to avoid losing highly trained staff on hospital transfers. CCPs are able to provide all of the care that PCPs and ACPs provide. That being said, CCPs significantly lack practical experience with advanced skills such as IV initiation, peripheral access to cardiovascular system for fluid and drug administration, advanced airway, and many other techniques. Where an PCP and ACP may run 40–50 medical codes per year a CCP may run 1–2 in an entire career. IV/IO starts are nearly non-existent in the field and for this reason CCPs are required to attend nearly double the amount of time in classroom situations or in hospital to keep current. In addition to this they are trained for other skills such as medication infusion pumps, mechanical ventilation and arterial line monitoring. CCPs often work in fixed and rotary wing aircraft when the weather permits and staff are available, but systems such as the Toronto EMS Critical Care Transport Program work in land ambulances. ORNGE Transport operates both land and aircraft in Ontario. In British Columbia, CCPs work primarily in aircraft with a dedicated Critical Care Transport crew in Trail for long-distance transfers and a regular CCP street crew stationed in South Vancouver that often also performs medevacs, when necessary.

Training

Paramedic training in Canada varies regionally; for example, the training may be eight months (British Columbia) or two to four years (Ontario, Alberta) in length. The nature of training and how it is regulated, like actual paramedic practice, varies from province to province.

Ireland

Emergency Medical Technician is a legally defined title in the Republic of Ireland based on the standard set down by the Pre-Hospital Emergency Care Council (PHECC). Emergency Medical Technician is the entry-level standard of practitioner for employment within the ambulance service. Currently, EMTs are authorised to work on non-emergency ambulances only as the standard for emergency (999) calls is a minimum of a two-paramedic crew. EMTs are a vital part of the voluntary and auxiliary services where a practitioner must be on board any ambulance in the process of transporting a patient to hospital.

PHECC Responder Levels		
Responder Title	**Abbr**	**Level of Care**
CARDIAC FIRST RESPONDER	**CFR**	Trained in BLS with emphasis on CPR and the Automated External Defibrillator
OCCUPATIONAL FIRST AIDER	**OFA**	Trained as CFR with additional training in management of bleeding, fractures etc. particularly in the workplace
EMERGENCY FIRST RESPONDER	**EFR**	Extensive first aid and BLS training with introduction to Oxygen therapy and assisting practitioners with care

PHECC Pract Emergency Medical Technician itioner Levels		
Practitioner Title	Abbr	Level of Care
EMERGENCY MEDICAL TECHNICIAN	EMT	Entry-level EMS Healthcare professional. Trained in BLS, Anatomy/Physiology, Pathophysiology, Pharmacology, ECG Monitoring, advanced Airway management (Supraglottic Airways) and Spinal Immobilization
PARAMEDIC	P	Emergency Ambulance Practitioner. Trained in advanced Pharmacology, advanced Airway management etc.
ADVANCED PARAMEDIC	AP	Trained to Paramedic level plus IV & IO access, a wide range of Medications, tracheal intubation, Manual Defib etc.

United Kingdom

Emergency Medical Technician is a term that has existed for many years in the United Kingdom. Some National Health Service ambulance services are running EMT conversion courses for staff who were trained by the Institute of Healthcare Development (IHCD) as Ambulance Technicians and Assistant Ambulance Practitioners. Ambulance trusts such as the London Ambulance Service and the North West Ambulance Service are in the process of converting existing Ambulance Technicians into Emergency Medical Technician grades 1, 2, 3 or 4, based on their level of experience; in many cases providing a similar level of care to that of a Paramedic.

Emergency Medical Technicians are still widely deployed in private ambulance companies with IHCD NHS trained Emergency Technicians being particularly sought after. There also many newer EMT training courses available. IHCD Ambulance Technicians and Assistant Ambulance Practitioners still exist within other UK ambulance services with Emergency Care Assistants employed in some areas as support, however, this grade of staff is now being phased out and replaced with a much lower qualified Emergency care assistants. The exception to this is the East of England Ambulance Service, who have actively stopped training Emergency Care Assistants, and is upskill training them to Emergency Medical Technician level. With the intention being to convert EMTs to Paramedics, thus up-skilling the entire workforce.

Examples of skills that may be had by an Emergency Medical Technician in the UK are:

- Administration of selected drugs (usually not IV Medications)

- Intermediate life support, including manual defibrillation and superglottic airway adjuncts

- Ability to discharge patient to different care pathways

- IV Cannulation (usually hospital EMT skill).

United States

History

The concept of modern-day Emergency Medical Services (EMS) care is widely noted to begin with the academic paper, "Accidental Death and Disability: The Neglected Disease of Modern Society", (or "White Paper") in 1966, according to EMS textbooks and relevant academia in the field. This paper detailed the statistics of highway accidents resulting in injury and death in the mid-1960s, as well as other causes of injury and death, and used the statistics to confirm that reform was needed in the United States, especially concerning public education and the amount of CPR and BLS/First Aid training received by police officers, firefighters, and ambulance services at the time.

The EMT program in the United States began as part of the "Alexandria Plan" in the early 1970s, in addition to a growing issue with injuries associated with car accidents. Emergency medicine (EM) as a medical specialty is relatively young. Prior to the 1960s and 1970s, hospital emergency departments were generally staffed by physicians on staff at the hospital on a rotating basis, among them general surgeons, internists, psychiatrists, and dermatologists. Physicians in training (interns and residents), foreign medical graduates and sometimes nurses also staffed the Emergency Department (ED). EM was born as a specialty in order to fill the time commitment required by physicians on staff to work in the increasingly chaotic emergency departments of the time. During this period, groups of physicians began to emerge who had left their respective practices in order to devote their work completely to the ED. The first of such groups was headed by Dr. James DeWitt Mills who, along with four associate physicians; Dr. Chalmers A. Loughridge, Dr. William Weaver, Dr. John McDade, and Dr. Steven Bednar at Alexandria Hospital, VA established 24/7 year-round emergency care which became known as the "Alexandria Plan". It was not until the establishment of American College of Emergency Physicians (ACEP), the recognition of emergency medicine training programs by the AMA and the AOA, and in 1979 a historical vote by the American Board of Medical Specialties that EM became a recognized medical specialty. The nation's first EMT's were from the Alexandria plan working as Emergency Care Technicians serving in the Alexandria Hospital Emergency Room. The training for these technicians was modeled after the established "Physician Assistant" training program and later restructured to meet the basic needs for emergency pre-hospital care. On June 24, 2011, The Alexandria Hospital Celebrated the 50th Anniversary of the Alexandria Plan. In attendance were three of the nation's first ECTs/EMTs: David Stover, Larry Jackson, and Kenneth Weaver.

Certification

In the United States, EMTs are certified according to their level of training. Individual states set their own standards of certification (or licensure, in some cases) and all EMT training must meet the minimum requirements as set by the National Highway Traffic

Safety Administration's (NHTSA) standards for curriculum. The National Registry of Emergency Medical Technicians (NREMT) is a private organization which offers certification exams based on NHTSA education guidelines and has been around since the 1970s. Currently, NREMT exams are used by 46 states as the sole basis for certification at one or more EMT certification levels. A NREMT exam consists of skills and patient assessments as well as a written portion.

In order to apply for the NREMT Certification applicants must be 18 years of age or older. A few states allow 16- and 17-year olds. Applicants must also successfully complete a state-approved EMT course that meets or exceeds the NREMT Standards within the past 2 years. Those applying for the NREMT Certification must also complete a state-approved EMT psychomotor exam.

The Veteran Emergency Medical Technician Support Act of 2013, H.R. 235 in the 113th United States Congress, would amend the Public Health Service Act to direct the Secretary of Health and Human Services to establish a demonstration program for states with a shortage of emergency medical technicians to streamline state requirements and procedures to assist veterans who completed military EMT training while serving in the Armed Forces to meet state EMT certification and licensure requirements. The bill passed in the United States House of Representatives, but has not yet been voted on in the United States Senate.

Levels

The NHTSA recognizes four levels of Emergency Medical Technician:

- EMR (Emergency Medical Responder)
- EMT (Emergency Medical Technician)
- AEMT (Advanced Emergency Medical Technician)
- Paramedic

Some states also recognize the Advanced Practice Paramedic or Critical Care Paramedic level as a state-specific licensure above that of the Paramedic. These Critical Care Paramedics generally perform high acuity transports that require skills outside the scope of a standard paramedic. In addition, EMTs can seek out specialty certifications such as Wilderness EMT, Wilderness Paramedic, Tactical EMT, and Flight Paramedic.

Transition to New Levels

In 2009, the NREMT posted information about a transition to a new system of levels for emergency care providers developed by the NHTSA with the National EMS Scope of Practice project. By 2014, these "new" levels will replace the fragmented system found around the United States. The new classification will include Emergency

Medical Responder (replacing first responder), Emergency Medical Technician (replacing EMT-Basic), Advanced Emergency Medical Technician (replacing EMT-Intermediate/85), and Paramedic (replacing EMT-Intermediate/99 and EMT-Paramedic). Education requirements in transitioning to the new levels are substantially similar.

EMR

EMR (Emergency Medical Responder) is the first, most basic level of EMS. EMRs, many of whom are volunteers, provide basic, immediate lifesaving care including bleeding control, manual stabilization of extremity fractures and suspected cervical spine injuries, eye irrigation, taking vital signs, supplemental oxygen administration, oral suctioning, positive pressure ventilation with a bag valve mask, cardio-pulmonary resuscitation (CPR), automated external defibrillator (AED) usage, assisting in a normal childbirth, and administration of certain basic medications such as epinephrine auto-injectors and oral glucose. Due to the opioid crisis, an increasing number of EMRs are now being trained in and allowed to administer intranasal naloxone. An EMR can assume care for a patient while more advanced resources are on the way, and then can assist EMTs and Paramedics when they arrive. Training requirements and treatment protocols vary from area to area.

EMT

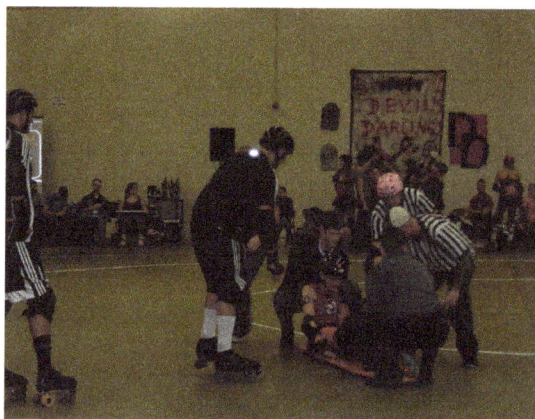

EMTs tend to a woman with a spiral fracture at a roller derby bout.

EMT is the next level of EMS. The procedures and skills allowed at this level include all EMR skills as well as nasopharyngeal airway, pulse oximetry, glucometry, splinting, use of a cervical collar, traction splinting, complicated childbirth delivery, and medication administration (such as epinephrine auto-injectors, oral glucose gel, aspirin (ASA), nitroglycerin, and albuterol). Some areas may add to the scope of practice for EMT's, including intranasal nalaxone administration, use of mechanical CPR devices, administration of intramuscular epinephrine and glucagon, insertion of additional airway devices, and CPAP. Training requirements and treatment protocols vary from area to area.

Advanced EMT

Advanced EMT is the levels of training between EMT and Paramedic. They can provide limited advanced life support (ALS) care including obtaining intravenous/intraosseous access, use of advanced airway devices, limited medication administration, and basic cardiac monitoring.

Paramedic

Paramedics, represents the highest level of EMT, and in general, the highest level of pre-hospital medical provider, though some areas utilize physicians as providers on air ambulances or as a ground provider. Paramedics perform a variety of medical procedures such as endotracheal intubation, fluid resuscitation, drug administration, obtaining intravenous access, cardiac monitoring (continuous and 12-lead), cardioversion, transcutaneous pacing, cricothyrotomy, manual defibrillation, chest needle decompression, and other advanced procedures and assessments.

Staffing Levels

An ambulance with only EMTs is considered a Basic Life Support (BLS) unit, an ambulance utilizing AEMTs is dubbed an Intermediate Life Support (ILS), or limited Advanced Life Support (LALS) unit, and an ambulance with Paramedics is dubbed an Advanced Life Support (ALS) unit. Some states allow ambulance crews to contain a mix of crews levels (e.g. an EMT and a Paramedic or an AEMT and a Paramedic) to staff ambulances and operate at the level of the highest trained provider. There is nothing stopping supplemental crew members to be of a certain certification, though (e.g. if an ALS ambulance is required to have two Paramedics, then it is acceptable to have two Paramedics and an EMT). An emergency vehicle with only EMRs or a combination of both EMRs and EMTs is still dubbed a Basic Life Support (BLS) unit. An EMR must be overseen by an EMT or higher to work on an ambulance.

Education and Training

EMT training programs for certification vary greatly from course to course, provided that each course at least meets local and national requirements. In the United States, EMR's receive at least 40–80 hours of classroom training, EMTs receive at least 120–180 hours of classroom training. AEMTs generally have 200–500 hours of training, and Paramedics are trained for 1,000–1,800 hours or more. In addition, a minimum number of continuing education (CE) hours are required to maintain certification. For example, to maintain NREMT certification, EMTs must obtain at least 48 hours of additional education and either complete a 24-hour refresher course or complete an additional 24 hours of CEs that would cover, on an hour by hour basis, the same topics as the refresher course would. Recertification for other levels follows a similar pattern.

EMT training programs vary greatly in calendar length (number of days or months). For example, fast track programs are available for EMTs that are completed in two weeks by holding class for 8 to 12 hours a day for at least two weeks. Other training programs are months long, or up to 2 years for Paramedics in an associate degree program. In addition to each level's didactic education, clinical rotations may also be required (especially for levels above EMT). Similar in a sense to medical school clinical rotations, EMT students are required to spend a required amount of time in an ambulance and on a variety of hospital services (e.g. obstetrics, emergency medicine, surgery, psychiatry) in order to complete a course and become eligible for the certification exam. The number of clinical hours for both time in an ambulance and time in the hour vary depending on local requirements, the level the student is obtaining, and the amount of time it takes the student to show competency. EMT training programs take place at numerous locations, such as universities, community colleges, technical schools, hospitals or EMS academies. Every state in the United States has an EMS lead agency or state office of emergency medical services that regulates and accredits EMT training programs. Most of these offices have web sites to provide information to the public and individuals who are interested in becoming an EMT.

Medical Direction

In the United States, an EMT's actions in the field are governed by state regulations, local regulations, and by the policies of their EMS organization. The development of these policies are guided by a physician medical director, often with the advice of a medical advisory committee.

In California, for example, each county's Local Emergency Medical Service Agency (LEMSA) issues a list of standard operating procedures or protocols, under the supervision of the California Emergency Medical Services Authority. These procedures often vary from county to county based on local needs, levels of training and clinical experiences. New York State has similar procedures, whereas a regional medical-advisory council ("REMAC") determines protocols for one or more counties in a geographical section of the state.

Treatments and procedures administered by Paramedics fall under one of two categories, off-line medical orders (standing orders) or on-line medical orders. On-line medical orders refers to procedures that must be explicitly approved by a base hospital physician or registered nurse through voice communication (generally by phone or radio) and are generally rare or high risk procedures (e.g. rapid sequence induction or cricothyrotomy). In addition, when multiple levels can perform the same procedure (e.g. AEMT-Critical Care and Paramedics in New York), a procedure can be both an on-line and a standing order depending on the level of the provider. Since no set of protocols can cover every patient situation, many systems work with protocols as guidelines and not "cook book" treatment plans. Finally, systems also have policies in place to handle medical direction when communication failures happen or in disaster situations. The NHTSA curriculum is the foundation Standard of Care for EMS providers in the US.

Employment

EMTs and Paramedics are employed in varied settings, mainly the prehospital environment such as in EMS, fire, and police agencies. They can also be found in positions ranging from hospital and health care settings, to industrial and entertainment positions. The prehospital environment is loosely divided into non-emergency (e.g. patient transport) and emergency (9-1-1 calls) services, but many ambulance services and EMS agencies operate both non-emergency and emergency care.

In many places across the United States, it is not uncommon for the primary employer of EMRs, EMTs, and Paramedics to be the fire department, with the fire department providing the primary emergency medical system response including "first responder" fire apparatus, as well as ambulances. In other locations, such as Boston, Massachusetts, emergency medical services are provided by a separate, or "third-party", municipal government emergency agency (e.g. Boston EMS). In still other locations, emergency medical services are provided by volunteer agencies. College and university campuses may provide emergency medical responses on their own campus using students.

In some states of the US, many EMS agencies are run by Independent Non-Profit Volunteer First Aid Squads that are their own corporations set up as separate entities from fire departments. In this environment, volunteers are hired to fill certain blocks of time to cover emergency calls. These volunteers have the same state certification as their paid counterparts.

Pre-hospital Emergency Medicine

Pre-hospital emergency medicine (abbreviated PHEM) is a medical speciality which focuses on caring for seriously ill or injured patients before they reach hospital, and during emergency transfer to hospital or between hospitals. It is primarily a subspecialty of emergency medicine, but may also be practised by physicians from other acute specialties such as anaesthesia, intensive care medicine and acute medicine.

Practitioners in PHEM are usually well-integrated with local emergency medical services, and are dispatched together with emergency medical technicians or paramedics where potentially life-threatening trauma or illness is suspected that may benefit from immediate specialist medical treatment. This may involve travelling by car or air ambulance to the site.

In the UK, PHEM was recognised as a subspecialty of emergency medicine and anaesthetics in July 2011 by the General Medical Council.

Pediatric Emergency Medicine

Pediatric emergency medicine (PEM) is a medical subspecialty of both pediatrics and emergency medicine. It involves the care of undifferentiated, unscheduled children with acute illnesses or injuries that require immediate medical attention. While not usually providing long-term or continuing care, pediatric emergency doctors undertake the necessary investigations and interventions to diagnose patients in the acute phase, to liaise with physicians from other specialities, and to resuscitate and stabilize children who are seriously ill or injured. Pediatric emergency physicians generally practice in hospital emergency departments.

Training

United States of America

Pediatric emergency physicians in the United States take one of two routes of training; one can do a pediatrics residency (3 years) followed by a pediatric emergency medicine fellowship (3 years), or an emergency medicine residency (3-4 years) followed by a pediatric emergency medicine fellowship. Majority of practicing PEM doctors take the former route. There are currently 52 PEM fellowship programs with 177 total spots in the United States. A survey published in 2009 found PEM physicians report high satisfaction levels, above those of doctors in all other specialties. Per doximity, pediatric emergency physicians in the U.S. made an average of $273,683 in 2014.

Canada

In Canada, aspiring paediatric emergency physicians must first complete a Doctor of Medicine (M.D.) and then apply to a paediatrics or emergency medicine residency program, both of which last on average five years. Residents, however, will not complete the entire residency program as they will, upon starting their final year of residency, switch to the other residency program in order to receive training in both specialties. This switch usually extends the length of the residency by a few years. As such, the residency program in its entirety usually has a length of about 6 years and leads to certification by the Royal College of Physicians and Surgeons of Canada.

Many institutions, such as McGill University, Université de Montréal, Université de Sherbrooke, and Université Laval in the province of Quebec, offer this residency program in collaboration with various hospital training centres. Other Canadian universities, such as University of Toronto, University of Ottawa, University of Calgary, University of Saskatchewan, and University of British Columbia, also offer post-graduate medical programs in emergency medicine and paediatrics.

Another general certification program is available for family physicians. Upon completing a two-year residency in family medicine, one has the possibility of completing a third year of residency in the emergency medicine enhanced skills program. Certification is awarded by the College of Family Physicians of Canada and allows family practitioners to work as emergency physicians in most emergency departments across Canada. The specialty training of family physicians allows them to treat patients of all ages affected by almost any type of disease. In that sense, family physicians who hold the emergency medicine certification may work with paediatric patients.

Diving Medicine

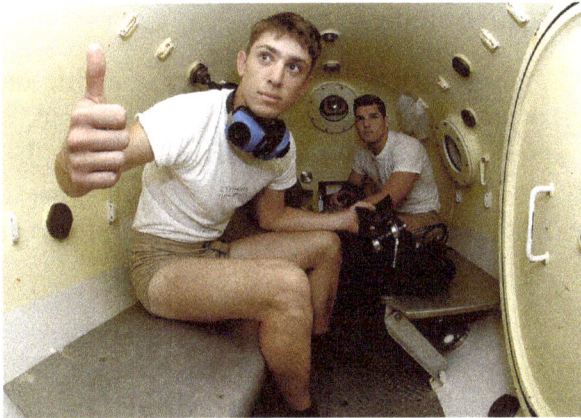

A recompression chamber is used to treat some diving disorders,
and for training divers to recognise the symptoms.

Diving medicine, also called undersea and hyperbaric medicine (UHB), is the diagnosis, treatment and prevention of conditions caused by humans entering the undersea environment. It includes the effects on the body of pressure on gases, the diagnosis and treatment of conditions caused by marine hazards and how relationships of a diver's fitness to dive affect a diver's safety.

Hyperbaric medicine is a corollary field associated with diving, since recompression in a hyperbaric chamber is used as a treatment for two of the most significant diving-related illnesses, decompression sickness and arterial gas embolism.

Diving medicine deals with medical research on issues of diving, the prevention of diving disorders, treatment of diving accidents and diving fitness. The field includes the effect of breathing gases and their contaminants under high pressure on the human body and the relationship between the state of physical and psychological health of the diver and safety.

In diving accidents it is common for multiple disorders to occur together and interact with each other, both causatively and as complications.

Diving medicine is a branch of occupational medicine and sports medicine, and an important part of diver education.

Range and Scope of Diving Medicine

The scope of diving medicine must necessarily include conditions that are specifically connected with the activity of diving, and not found in other contexts, but this categorization excludes almost everything, leaving only deep water blackout, isobaric counterdiffusion and high pressure nervous syndrome. A more useful grouping is conditions that are associated with exposure to variations of ambient pressure. These conditions are largely shared by aviation and space medicine. Further conditions associated with diving and other aquatic and outdoor activities are commonly included in books which are aimed at the diver, rather than the specialist medical practitioner, as they are useful background to diver first aid training.

The scope of knowledge necessary for a practitioner of diving medicine includes the medical conditions associated with diving and their treatment, physics and physiology relating to the underwater and pressurised environment, the standard operating procedures and equipment used by divers which can influence the development and management of these conditions, and the specialised equipment used for treatment.

Scope of Knowledge for Diving Medicine

The ECHM-EDTC Educational and Training Standards for Diving and Hyperbaric Medicine (2011) specify the following scope of knowledge for Diving Medicine:

• Physiology and pathology of diving and hyperbaric exposure. 　○ Hyperbaric physics 　○ Diving related physiology 　○ Hyperbaric pathophysiology of immersion 　○ Pathophysiology of decompression 　○ A brief introduction to acute dysbaric disorders • Diving technology and safety 　○ Basic safety planning 　○ Compressed air work 　○ Diving procedures 　○ Diving tables and computers 　○ Regulations and standards for diving	• Fitness to dive 　○ Fitness to dive criteria and contraindications for divers, compressed air workers and HBOT chamber personnel • Diving accidents 　○ Diving incidents and accidents 　○ Emergency medical support with no chamber on site

Scope of Knowledge for Hyperbaric Medicine

The ECHM-EDTC Educational and Training Standards for Diving and Hyperbaric Medicine (2011) specify the following scope of knowledge for Hyperbaric Medicine additional to that for Diving medicine:

- Physiology and pathology of diving and hyperbaric exposure.

    o HBO-Basics - effects of hyperbaric oxygen - physiology and pathology

- Clinical HBO

    o Chamber technique (multiplace, monoplace, transport chambers, wet recompression)

    o Mandatory indications

    o HBO General basic treatment (nursing)

    o HBO Diagnostic, monitoring and therapeutic devices in chambers

    o Risk assessment, incidents monitoring and safety plan in HBO chambers

    o HBO Safety regulations

Diagnostics

The signs and symptoms of diving disorders may present during a dive, on surfacing, or up to several hours after a dive. Divers have to breathe a gas which is at the same pressure as their surroundings, which can be much greater than on the surface. The ambient pressure underwater increases by 1 standard atmosphere (100 kPa) for every 10 metres (33 ft) of depth.

The principal conditions are: decompression illness (which covers decompression sickness and arterial gas embolism); nitrogen narcosis; high pressure nervous syndrome; oxygen toxicity; and pulmonary barotrauma (burst lung). Although some of these may occur in other settings, they are of particular concern during diving activities.

The disorders are caused by breathing gas at the high pressures encountered at depth, and divers will often breathe a gas mixture different from air to mitigate these effects. Nitrox, which contains more oxygen and less nitrogen is commonly used as a breathing gas to reduce the risk of decompression sickness at recreational depths (up to about 40 metres (130 ft)). Helium may be added to reduce the amount of nitrogen and oxygen in the gas mixture when diving deeper, to reduce the effects of narcosis and to avoid the risk of oxygen toxicity. This is complicated at depths beyond about 150 metres (500 ft), because a helium–oxygen mixture (heliox) then causes high pressure nervous syndrome. More exotic mixtures such as hydreliox, a hydrogen–helium–oxygen mixture, are used at extreme depths to counteract this.

Decompression Sickness

Decompression sickness (DCS) occurs when gas, which has been breathed under high pressure and dissolved into the body tissues, forms bubbles as the pressure is reduced on ascent from a dive. The results may range from pain in the joints where the bubbles form to blockage of an artery leading to damage to the nervous system, paralysis or death. While bubbles can form anywhere in the body, DCS is most frequently observed in the shoulders, elbows, knees, and ankles. Joint pain occurs in about 90% of DCS cases reported to the U.S. Navy, with neurological symptoms and skin manifestations each present in 10% to 15% of cases. Pulmonary DCS is very rare in divers.

Pulmonary Barotrauma and Arterial Gas Embolism

If the breathing gas in a diver's lungs cannot freely escape during an ascent, the lungs may be expanded beyond their compliance, and the lung tissues may rupture, causing pulmonary barotrauma (PBT). The gas may then enter the arterial circulation producing arterial gas embolism (AGE), with effects similar to severe decompression sickness. Gas bubbles within the arterial circulation can block the supply of blood to any part of the body, including the brain, and can therefore manifest a vast variety of symptoms.

Nitrogen Narcosis

Nitrogen narcosis is caused by the pressure of dissolved gas in the body and produces impairment to the nervous system. This results in alteration to thought processes and a decrease in the diver's ability to make judgements or calculations. It can also decrease motor skills, and worsen performance in tasks requiring manual dexterity. As depth increases, so does the pressure and hence the severity of the narcosis. The effects may vary widely from individual to individual, and from day to day for the same diver. Because of the perception-altering effects of narcosis, a diver may not be aware of the symptoms, but studies have shown that impairment occurs nevertheless.

High Pressure Nervous Syndrome

Helium is the least narcotic of all gases, and divers may use breathing mixtures containing a proportion of helium for dives exceeding about 40 metres (130 ft) deep. In the 1960s it was expected that helium narcosis would begin to become apparent at depths of 300 metres (1,000 ft). However, it was found that different symptoms, such as tremors, occurred at shallower depths around 150 metres (500 ft). This became known as high pressure nervous syndrome, and its effects are found to result from both the absolute depth and the speed of descent. Although the effects vary from person to person, they are stable and reproducible for the individual.

Oxygen Toxicity

Although oxygen is essential to life, in concentrations significantly greater than normal it becomes toxic, overcoming the body's natural defences (antioxidants), and causing cell death in any part of the body. The lungs and brain are particularly affected by high partial pressures of oxygen, such as are encountered in diving. The body can tolerate partial pressures of oxygen around 0.5 bars (50 kPa; 7.3 psi) indefinitely, and up to 1.4 bars (140 kPa; 20 psi) for many hours, but higher partial pressures rapidly increase the chance of the most dangerous effect of oxygen toxicity, a convulsion resembling an epileptic seizure. Susceptibility to oxygen toxicity varies dramatically from person to person, and to a smaller extent from day to day for the same diver. Prior to convulsion, several symptoms may be present – most distinctly that of an aura.

Treatments

Treatment of diving disorders depends on the specific disorder or combination of disorders, but two treatments are commonly associated with first aid and definitive treatment where diving is involved. These are first aid oxygen administration at high concentration, which is seldom contraindicated, and generally recommended as a default option in diving accidents where there is any significant probability of hypoxia, and hyperbaric oxygen therapy, which is the definitive treatment for most incidences of decompression illness. Hyperbaric treatment using other breathing gases is also used for treatment of decompression sickness if HBO is inadequate.

Oxygen Therapy

The administration of oxygen as a medical intervention is common in diving medicine, both for first aid and for longer term treatment.

Recompression and Hyperbaric Oxygen Therapy

Recompression treatment in a hyperbaric chamber was initially used as a life-saving tool to treat decompression sickness in caisson workers and divers who stayed too long at depth and developed decompression sickness. Now, it is a highly specialized treatment modality that has been found to be effective in the treatment of many conditions where the administration of oxygen under pressure has been found to be beneficial. Studies have shown it to be quite effective in some 13 indications approved by the Undersea and Hyperbaric Medical Society.

Hyperbaric oxygen treatment is generally preferred when effective, as it is usually a more efficient and lower risk method of reducing symptoms of decompression illness, but in some cases recompression to pressures where oxygen toxicity is unacceptable may be required to eliminate the bubbles in the tissues in severe cases of decompression illness.

Education and Registration of Practitioners

Specialist training in underwater and hyperbaric medicine is available from several institutions, and registration is possible both with professional associations and governmental registries.

Education

NOAA/UHMS Physicians Training Course in Diving Medicine

> This course has been presented since 1977, and has been influenced by internationally accepted training objectives recommended by the Diving Medical Advisory Committee, the European Diving Technology Committee, and the European Committee for Hyperbaric Medicine. The course is designed for qualified medical practitioners, but may be useful to others who work in the field of diving safety and operations.

The course is to train physicians to recognize and treat diving medical emergencies. Subject matter includes:

- Basic physics and physiology of the hyperbaric environment:
    - the laws and principles;
    - the differences between hyperbaric and hypobaric pressure;
    - hyperbaric gases and their effects under pressure;
    - links between the physiological effects of the hyperbaric environment and the pathology of the disease

- Basic decompression theory:
    - historical development to current concepts
    - factors affecting decompression safety including acceptable risks and thermal issues
    - distinguish decompression sickness from barotrauma and arterial gas embolism;

- Dive computer theories and types, and comparison to dive tables

- Introduction to commercial diving and comparison to recreational and technical diving, including differences in procedures, equipment, and diver categories

- The clinical application of hyperbaric oxygen therapy and the treatment tables used;

- Participation in surface-supplied diving operation and hyperbaric chamber operations;

- Components, types, operational and safety hazards associated with hyperbaric chambers;

- Diving-related conditions resulting from the effects of long-term effects of diving, flying after diving, altitude, thermal conditions, age and gender

- Neurologic assessment on a diver with signs and/or symptoms of DCI

- Medical and fitness standards for diving, including:

  o contraindications for both commercial and recreational divers

  o differences in medical standards for recreational versus occupational diving communities

  o legal implications for approving and denying fitness to dive in an occupational setting

  o approaches for determining the safety of prescription and OTC medications used by divers

Fellowship in Undersea and Hyperbaric Medicine

The Accreditation Council for Graduate Medical Education (ACGME) and the American Osteopathic Association (AOA) offer 12 month programs in undersea and hyperbaric medicine associated with ACGME or AOA accredited programs in emergency medicine, family medicine, internal medicine, occupational medicine, preventive medicine, or anesthesiology.

ECHM-EDTC Educational and Training Standards for Physicians in Diving and Hyperbaric Medicine

The standard drawn up jointly by the European Committee for Hyperbaric Medicine and the European Diving Technical Committee defines job descriptions for several levels of diving and hyperbaric physician: Education and assessment to these standards may be provided by institutions of higher education under the leadership of a Level 3 Hyperbaric Medicine Expert as defined below. Certificates of competence may be issued by a nationally accredited institution or an internationally acknowledged agency, and periodic recertification is required.

Level 1. *Medical Examiner of Divers* (MED) minimum 28 teaching hours.

- The MED must be competent to perform the assessments of medical fitness to dive of occupational and recreational divers and compressed air workers, except the assessment of medical fitness to resume diving after major decompression incidents.

Level 2D. *Diving Medicine Physician* (DMP) minimum 80 teaching hours.

- A DMP must be competent to perform the initial and all other assessments of medical fitness to dive of working and recreational divers or compressed air workers, and manage diving accidents and advise diving contractors and others on diving medicine and physiology (with the backup of a diving medical expert or consultant).

- A DMP should have knowledge in relevant aspects of occupational health, but is not required to be a certified specialist in occupational medicine.

- A DMP should have certified skills and basic practical experience in assessment of medical fitness to dive, management of diving accidents, safety planning for professional diving operations, advanced life support, acute trauma care and general wound care.

Level 2H. *Hyperbaric Medicine Physician* (HMP) minimum 120 teaching hours

- An HMP will be responsible for hyperbaric treatment sessions (with the backup of a hyperbaric medicine expert or consultant)

- An HMP should have appropriate experience in anaesthesia and intensive care in order to manage the HBO patients, but is not required to be a certified specialist in anaesthesia and intensive care.

- An HMP must be competent to assess and manage clinical patients for hyperbaric oxygen therapy treatment.

Level 3. *Hyperbaric medicine expert or consultant (hyperbaric and diving medicine)* is a physician who has been assessed as competent to:

- manage a hyperbaric facility (HBO centre) or the medical and physiological aspects of complex diving activities.

- manage research programs on diving medicine.

- supervise a team of HBO doctors and personnel, health professionals and others.

- teach relevant aspects of hyperbaric medicine and physiology to all members of staff.

Gesellschaft für Tauch- und Überdruckmedizin e. V.

> *Society for Diving and Hyperbaric medicine*
> German standards for education and assessment of diving medical practitioners are similar to the ECHM-EDTC Standards and are controlled by the Gesellschaft für Tauch- und Überdruckmedizin e. V.. They include Medical Examiner of Divers, Diving Medicine Physician, Hyperbaric Medicine Physician, Chief Hyperbaric Medicine Physician and Hyperbaric Medicine Consultant.

Schweizerische Gesellschaft für Unterwasser- und Hyperbarmedizin

> *Swiss Society for underwater and hyperbaric medicine.*
> Swiss standards for education and assessment of diving medical practitioners are controlled by the Schweizerische Gesellschaft für Unterwasser- und Hyperbarmedizin. They include Medical Examiner of Divers, Diving Medicine Physician and Hyperbaric Medicine Physician.

Österreichische Gesellschaft für Tauch- und Hyperbarmedizin

> *Austrian Society for Diving and Hyperbaric medicine.*
> Austrian standards for education and assessment of diving medical practitioners are controlled by the Österreichische Gesellschaft für Tauch- und Hyperbarmedizin They include Medical Examiner of Divers, Diving Medicine Physician, Hyperbaric Medicine Physician, Chief Hyperbaric Medicine Physician and Hyperbaric Medicine Consultant.

Registration

The American Medical Association recognises the sub-speciality *Undersea and Hyperbaric Medicine* held by someone who is already Board Certified in some other speciality.

The South African Department of Labour registers two levels of *Diving Medical Practitioner*. Level 1 is qualified to conduct annual examinations and certification of medical fitness to dive, on commercial divers (equivalent to ECHM-EDTC Level 1. Medical Examiner of Divers), and Level 2 is qualified to provide medical advice to a diving contractor and hyperbaric treatment for diving injuries (equivalent to ECHM-EDTC Level 2D Diving Medicine Physician)

Australia has a four tier system: In 2007 there was no recognised equivalence with the European standard.

- GPs completing the first tier four- to five-day course on how to examine divers for 'fitness to dive' can then add their names to the SPUMS Diving Doctors List.

- GPs completing the second tier two-week diving medicine courses provided by the Royal Australian Navy and the Royal Adelaide Hospital, or the two-week course in Diving and Hyperbaric Medicine provided by the ANZ Hyperbaric Medicine Group, qualify to do commercial-diving medicals.

- The third tier is the SPUMS Diploma in Diving and Hyperbaric Medicine. The candidate must attend a two-week course, write a dissertation related to DHM and have the equivalent of six months' full-time experience working in a hyperbaric medicine unit.

- The fourth tier is the Certificate in Diving and Hyperbaric Medicine from the ANZ College of Anaesthetists.

Training of Divers and Support Staff in Relevant First Aid

Divers

A basic knowledge understanding of the causes, symptoms and first aid treatment of diving related disorders is part of the basic training for most recreational and professional divers, both to help the diver avoid the disorders, and to allow appropriate action in case of an incident resulting in injury.

Recreational Divers

A recreational diver has the same duty of care to other divers as any ordinary member of the public, and therefore there is no obligation to train recreational divers in first aid or other medical skills. Nevertheless, first aid is training is recommended by most, if not all, recreational diver training agencies.

Recreational diving instructors and divemasters, on the other hand, are to a greater or lesser extent responsible for the safety of divers under their guidance, and therefore are generally required to be trained and certified to some level of rescue and first aid competence, as defined in the relevant training standards of the certifying body. In many cases this includes certification in Cardiopulmonary resuscitation and Oxygen administration for diving accidents.

Professional Divers

Professional divers usually operate as members of a team with a duty of care for other members of the team. Divers are expected to act as standby divers for other members of the team and the duties of a standby diver include rescue attempts if the working diver gets into difficulties. Consequently, professional divers are generally required to be trained in rescue procedures appropriate to the modes of diving they are certified in, and to administer first aid in emergencies. The specific training, competence and registration for these skills varies, and may be specified by state or national legislation or by industry codes of practice.

Diving supervisors have a similar duty of care, and as they are responsible for operational planning and safety, generally are also expected to manage emergency procedures, including the first aid that may be required. The level of first aid training, competence and certification will generally take this into account.

- In South Africa, registered commercial and scientific divers must hold current certification in first aid at the national Level 1, with additional training in oxygen administration for diving accidents, and registered diving supervisors must hold Level 2 first aid certification.

- Offshore diving contractors frequently follow the IMCA recommendations.

Diver Medic

A diver medic is a member of a dive team who is trained in advanced first aid. A Diver Medic recognised by IMCA must be capable of administering First Aid and emergency treatment, and carrying out the directions of a doctor pending the arrival of more skilled medical aid, and therefore must be able to effectively communicate with a doctor who is not on site, and be familiar with diving procedures and compression chamber operation. The Diver Medic must also be able to assist the diving supervisor with decompression procedures provide advice as to when more specialised medical help should be requested, and must be fit to provide treatment in a hyperbaric chamber in an emergency, and must therefore hold a valid certificate of medical fitness to dive.

Training standards for Diver Medic are described in the IMCA Scheme for Recognition of Diver Medic Training.

History of Diving Medical Research

Timeline

- November 1992: The first examination for certification in Undersea Medicine by the American Board of Preventive Medicine.

- November 1999: The first examination for Undersea and Hyperbaric Medicine qualification.

Notable Researchers

• Arthur J. Bachrach	• Brian A. Hills
• Albert R. Behnke	• F. J. Keays
• Peter B. Bennett	• Christian J. Lambertsen
• Thomas E. Berghage	• Simon Mitchell
• Paul Bert	• Richard E. Moon
• George F. Bond	• František Novomeský
• Alf O. Brubakk	• John Rawlins (Royal Navy officer)
• Albert A. Bühlmann	• Charles Wesley Shilling
• Carl Edmonds	• Edward D. Thalmann
• William Paul Fife	• Richard D. Vann
• John Scott Haldane	• James Vorosmarti
• Robert William Hamilton, Jr.	• R. M. Wong
• Leonard Erskine Hill	• Robert D. Workman

Research Organisations

Defence and Civil Institute of Environmental Medicine

DCIEM is a combined military and civilian research organisation to research the operational needs of the Canadian Forces in all environments.

Divers Alert Network

The Divers Alert Network (DAN) is an international non-profit organization with regional branches supported by donations, grants, and membership dues, for assisting divers in need. The DAN Research department conducts significant medical research on recreational scuba diving safety, and the DAN Medicine Department provides support for divers worldwide to find answers to their diving medical questions.

Diving Diseases Research Centre

The Diving Diseases Research Centre (DDRC) is a British hyperbaric medical organisation located near Derriford Hospital in Plymouth, Devon. It is a registered charity and was established in 1980 to research the effects of diving on human physiology.

The main objective of DDRC is research into diving medicine. The Centre is also an education and training base providing diving medical, clinical and hyperbaric courses.

Diving Medical Advisory Committee

> DMAC is an independent committee with the purpose of providing advice about medical and safety aspects of commercial diving. They publish guidance notes about various aspects of diving and diving medical practice, and run a scheme for approval of courses in diving medicine.

European Committee for Hyperbaric Medicine

> The ECHM is an organisation to study and define indications for hyperbaric therapy, research and therapy protocols, standards for therapeutic and technical procedures, equipment and personnel, and related cost-benefit and cost-effectiveness criteria. It is a representative body with the European health authorities, and works toward cooperation among scientific organizations involved in the field of Diving and Hyperbaric Medicine.

Membership of the committee includes doctors practicing diving medicine in Northern Europe, representatives of relevant health authorities, medical representatives from relevant navies, and a diving safety officer nominated by the International Marine Contractors Association.

European Underwater and Baromedical Society

The European Underwater and Baromedical Society (EUBS) is a primary source of information for diving and hyperbaric medicine physiology worldwide. The organization was initially formed as the European Underwater and Biomedical Society in 1971.

National Board of Diving and Hyperbaric Medical Technology

The National Board of Diving and Hyperbaric Medical Technology (NBDHMT), formally known as the National Association of Diving Technicians, is a non-profit organization for the education and certification of qualified personnel in the fields of diving and hyperbaric medicine in the US.

- The Diver Medic Technician (DMT) program is designed to meet the specific medical care needs of commercial, professional and scientific divers that often work in geographic isolation. DMT's are specifically trained for the various diving hazards found at remote work sites. The curriculum covers a wide range of topics from barotrauma to treatment of decompression sickness.

- The Certified Hyperbaric Technologist (CHT) program is tailored to meet the specific safety and operational needs for biomedical devices within the department, and the necessary knowledge and skills to administer clinical treatment. The curriculum covers a wide range of topics including hyperbaric chamber operations to transcutaneous oxygen monitoring.

- The Certified Hyperbaric Registered Nurse (CHRN) program is a subspecialty for registered nurses, sometimes referred to as baromedical nurses.

Southern African Undersea and Hyperbaric Medical Association

SAUHMA is a voluntary association recognised as a Special Interest group by the Group Council of the South African Medical Association.

South Pacific Underwater Medicine Society

The South Pacific Underwater Medicine Society (SPUMS) is a primary source of information for diving and hyperbaric medicine physiology worldwide. The organisation supports the study of all aspects of underwater and hyperbaric medicine, provides information on underwater and hyperbaric medicine, publishes a medical journal and holds an annual conference.

SPUMS offers a post-graduate Diploma of Diving and Hyperbaric Medicine.

Undersea and Hyperbaric Medical Society

The Undersea and Hyperbaric Medical Society (UHMS) is a primary source of information for diving and hyperbaric medicine physiology worldwide.

Hyperbaric Medicine

Hyperbaric medicine is medical treatment in which an ambient pressure greater than sea level atmospheric pressure is a necessary component. The treatment comprises hyperbaric oxygen therapy (HBOT), the medical use of oxygen at an ambient pressure higher than atmospheric pressure, and therapeutic recompression for decompression illness, intended to reduce the injurious effects of systemic gas bubbles by physically reducing their size and providing improved conditions for elimination of bubbles and excess dissolved gas.

The equipment required for hyperbaric oxygen treatment consists of a pressure chamber, which may be of rigid or flexible construction, and a means of delivering 100% oxygen. Operation is performed to a predetermined schedule by trained personnel who monitor the patient and may adjust the schedule as required. HBOT found early use in the treatment of decompression sickness, and has also shown great effectiveness in treating conditions such as gas gangrene and carbon monoxide poisoning. More recent research has examined the possibility that it may also have value for other conditions such as cerebral palsy and multiple sclerosis, but no significant evidence has been found.

Therapeutic recompression is usually also provided in a hyperbaric chamber. It is the definitive treatment for decompression sickness and may also be used to treat arterial gas embolism caused by pulmonary barotrauma of ascent. In emergencies divers may sometimes be treated by in-water recompression if a chamber is not available and suitable diving equipment to reasonably secure the airway is available.

A number of hyperbaric treatment schedules have been published over the years for both therapeutic recompression and hyperbaric oxygen therapy for other conditions.

Scope

Hyperbaric medicine includes hyperbaric oxygen treatment, which is the medical use of oxygen at greater than atmospheric pressure to increase the availability of oxygen in the body; and therapeutic recompression, which involves increasing the ambient pressure on a person, usually a diver, to treat decompression sickness or an air embolism by eliminating bubbles that have formed within the body.

Medical Uses

In the United States the Undersea and Hyperbaric Medical Society, known as UHMS, lists approvals for reimbursement for certain diagnoses in hospitals and clinics. The following indications are approved (for reimbursement) uses of hyperbaric oxygen therapy as defined by the UHMS Hyperbaric Oxygen Therapy Committee:

- Air or gas embolism;

- Carbon monoxide poisoning;

    o Carbon monoxide poisoning complicated by cyanide poisoning;

- Central retinal artery occlusion;

- Clostridal myositis and myonecrosis (gas gangrene);

- Crush injury, compartment syndrome, and other acute traumatic ischemias;

- Decompression sickness;

- Enhancement of healing in selected problem wounds;.

    o Diabetically derived illness, such as short-term relief of diabetic foot,diabetic retinopathy, diabetic nephropathy;

- Exceptional blood loss (anemia);

- Idiopathic sudden sensorineural hearing loss;

- Intracranial abscess;

- Mucormycosis, especially rhinocerebral disease in the setting of diabetes mellitus;

- Necrotizing soft tissue infections (necrotizing fasciitis);

- Osteomyelitis (refractory);

- Delayed radiation injury (soft tissue and bony necrosis);

- Skin grafts and flaps (compromised);

- Thermal burns.

Evidence is insufficient as of 2013 to support its use in autism, cancer, diabetes, HIV/AIDS, Alzheimer's disease, asthma, Bell's palsy, cerebral palsy, depression, heart disease, migraines, multiple sclerosis, Parkinson's disease, spinal cord injury, sports injuries, or stroke. A Cochrane review published in 2016 has raised questions about the ethical basis for future clinical trials of hyperbaric oxygen therapy, in view of the increased risk of damage to the eardrum in children with autism spectrum disorders. Despite the lack of evidence, in 2015, the number of people utilizing this therapy has continued to rise.

Hearing Issues

There is limited evidence that hyperbaric oxygen therapy improves hearing in patients with sudden sensorineural hearing loss who present within two weeks of hearing loss. There is some indication that HBOT might improve tinnitus presenting in the same time frame.

Chronic Ulcers

HBOT in diabetic foot ulcers increased the rate of early ulcer healing but does not appear to provide any benefit in wound healing at long term follow-up. In particular, there was no difference in major amputation rate. For venous, arterial and pressure ulcers, no evidence was apparent that HBOT provides an improvement over standard treatment.

Radiation Injury

There is some evidence that HBOT is effective for late radiation tissue injury of bone and soft tissues of the head and neck. Some people with radiation injuries of the head, neck or bowel show an improvement in quality of life. Importantly, no such effect has been found in neurological tissues. The use of HBOT may be justified to selected patients and tissues, but further research is required to establish the best people to treat and timing of any HBO therapy.

Neuro-rehabilitation

There is tentative evidence for HBOT in traumatic brain injury. As of 2012 there is insufficient evidence to support its general use in TBI. In stroke HBOT does not show benefit. HBOT in multiple sclerosis has not shown benefit and routine use is not recommended.

A 2007 review of HBOT in cerebral palsy found no difference compared to the control group. Neuropsychological tests also showed no difference between HBOT and room air and based on caregiver report, those who received room air had significantly better mobility and social functioning. Children receiving HBOT were reported to experience seizures and the need for tympanostomy tubes to equalize ear pressure, though the incidence was not clear.

Cancer

In alternative medicine, hyperbaric medicine has been promoted as a treatment for cancer. A 2012 review article in the journal, *Targeted Oncology,* reports that "there is no evidence indicating that HBO neither acts as a stimulator of tumor growth nor as an enhancer of recurrence. On the other hand, there is evidence that implies that HBO might have tumor-inhibitory effects in certain cancer subtypes, and we thus strongly believe that we need to expand our knowledge on the effect and the mechanisms behind tumor oxygenation." However, a 2011 study by the American Cancer Society reported no evidence it is effective for this purpose.

Contraindications

The toxicology of the treatment has recently been reviewed by Ustundag *et al.* and its risk management is discussed by Christian R. Mortensen, in light of the fact that most hyperbaric facilities are managed by departments of anaesthesiology and some of their patients are critically ill.

The only absolute contraindication to hyperbaric oxygen therapy is untreated pneumothorax. The reason is concern that it can progress to tension pneumothorax, especially during the decompression phase of therapy, although treatment on oxygen-based tables may avoid that progression. The COPD patient with a large bleb represents a relative contraindication for similar reasons. Also, the treatment may raise the issue of Occupational health and safety (OHS), which has been encountered by the therapist.

Patients should not undergo HBO therapy if they are taking or have recently taken the following drugs:

- Doxorubicin (Adriamycin) – A chemotherapeutic drug. This drug has been shown to potentiate cytotoxicity during HBO therapy.

- Cisplatin – Also a chemotherapeutic drug.

- Disulfiram (Antabuse) – Used in the treatment of alcoholism.

- Mafenide acetate (Sulfamylon) – Suppresses bacterial infections in burn wounds

The following are relative contraindications -- *meaning that special consideration must be made by specialist physicians before HBO treatments begin:*

- Cardiac disease

- COPD with air trapping - can lead to pneumothorax during treatment.

- Upper respiratory infections – These conditions can make it difficult for the patient to equalise their ears or sinuses, which can result in what is termed ear or sinus squeeze.

- High fevers – In most cases the fever should be lowered before HBO treatment begins. Fevers may predispose to convulsions.

- Emphysema with CO_2 retention – This condition can lead to pneumothorax during HBO treatment due to rupture of an emphysematous bulla. This risk can be evaluated by x-ray.

- History of thoracic (chest) surgery – This is rarely a problem and usually not considered a contraindication. However, there is concern that air may be trapped in lesions that were created by surgical scarring. These conditions need to be evaluated prior to considering HBO therapy.

- Malignant disease: Cancers thrive in blood-rich environments but may be suppressed by high oxygen levels. HBO treatment of individuals who have cancer presents a problem, since HBO both increases blood flow via angiogenesis and also raises oxygen levels. Taking an anti-angiogenic supplement may provide a solution. A study by Feldemier, et al. and recent NIH funded study on Stem Cells by Thom, et al., indicate that HBO is actually beneficial in producing stem/progenitor cells and the malignant process is not accelerated.

- Middle ear barotrauma is always a consideration in treating both children and adults in a hyperbaric environment because of the necessity to equalise pressure in the ears.

Pregnancy is not a relative contraindication to hyperbaric oxygen treatments, although it may be for underwater diving. In cases where a pregnant woman has carbon monoxide poisoning there is evidence that lower pressure (2.0 ATA) HBOT treatments are not harmful to the fetus, and that the risk involved is outweighed by the greater risk of the untreated effects of CO on the fetus (neurologic abnormalities or death.) In pregnant patients, HBO therapy has been shown to be safe for the fetus when given at appropriate levels and "doses" (durations). In fact, pregnancy lowers the threshold for HBO treatment of carbon monoxide-exposed patients. This is due to the high affinity of fetal hemoglobin for CO.

Therapeutic Principles

The therapeutic consequences of HBOT and recompression result from multiple effects. The increased overall pressure is of therapeutic value in the treatment of decompression sickness and air embolism as it provides a physical means of reducing the volume of inert gas bubbles within the body; Exposure to this increased pressure is maintained for a period long enough to ensure that most of the bubble gas is dissolved back into the tissues, removed by perfusion and eliminated in the lungs. The improved concentration gradient for inert gas elimination (oxygen window) by using a high partial pressure of oxygen increases the rate of inert gas elimination in the treatment of decompression sickness. For many other conditions, the therapeutic principle of HBOT lies in its ability to drastically increase partial pressure of oxygen in the tissues of the body. The oxygen partial pressures achievable using HBOT are much higher than those achievable while breathing pure oxygen under normobaric conditions (i.e. at normal atmospheric pressure); A related effect is the increased oxygen transport capacity of the blood. Under normal atmospheric pressure, oxygen transport is limited by the oxygen binding capacity of hemoglobin in red blood cells and very little oxygen is transported by blood plasma. Because the hemoglobin of the red blood cells is almost saturated with oxygen under atmospheric pressure, this route of transport cannot be exploited any further. Oxygen transport by plasma, however is significantly increased using HBOT as the stimulus. Recent evidence suggests that exposure to hyperbaric oxygen (HBOT) mobilizes stem/progenitor cells from the bone marrow by a nitric oxide (NO) -dependent mechanism. This mechanism may account for the patient cases that indicate recovery of damaged organs and tissues with HBOT.

Hyperbaric Chambers

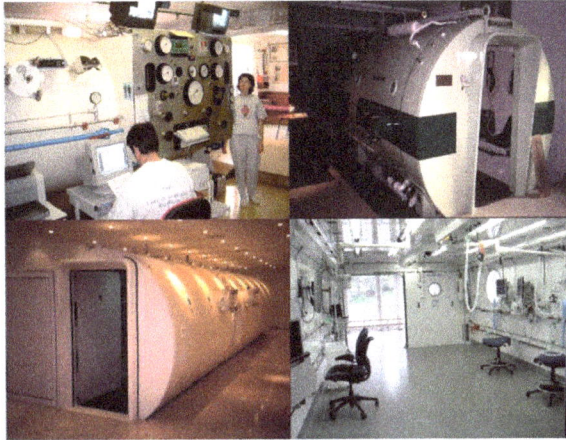

Multiplace hyperbaric chambers, showing control panel, monitoring facilities,
and different chamber sizes in Spanish facilities

Construction

The traditional type of hyperbaric chamber used for therapeutic recompression and
HBOT is a rigid shelled pressure vessel. Such chambers can be run at absolute pressures
typically about 6 bars (87 psi), 600,000 Pa or more in special cases. Navies, professional diving organizations, hospitals, and dedicated recompression facilities typically
operate these. They range in size from semi-portable, one-patient units to room-sized
units that can treat eight or more patients. The larger units may be rated for lower pressures if they are not primarily intended for treatment of diving injuries.

A rigid chamber may consist of:

- a pressure vessel that is generally made of steel or aluminium with the view
  ports (windows) made of acrylic;

- one or more human entry hatches—small and circular or wheel-in type hatches
  for patients on gurneys;

- the entry lock that allows human entry—a separate chamber with two hatches,
  one to the outside and one to the main chamber, which can be independently
  pressurized to allow patients to enter or exit the main chamber while it is still
  pressurized.

- a low volume medical or service airlock for medicines, instruments, and food;

- transparent ports or closed-circuit television that allows technicians and medical staff outside the chamber to monitor the patient inside the chamber;

- an intercom system allowing two-way communication;

- an optional carbon dioxide scrubber—consisting of a fan that passes the gas inside the chamber through a soda lime canister;

- a control panel outside the chamber to open and close valves that control air flow to and from the chamber, and regulate oxygen to hoods or masks;

- an over-pressure relief valve.

- a built-in breathing system (BIBS) to supply and exhaust treatment gas.

- a fire suppression system.

Flexible monoplace chambers are available ranging from collapsible flexible aramid fiber-reinforced chambers which can be disassembled for transport via truck or SUV, with a maximum working pressure of 2 bar above ambient complete with BIBS allowing full oxygen treatment schedules. to portable, air inflated "soft" chambers that can operate at between 0.3 and 0.5 bars (4.4 and 7.3 psi) above atmospheric pressure with no supplemental oxygen, and longitudinal zipper closure.

Hard chambers and soft chambers are not equivalent in efficacy and safety as they are different in many aspects.

Oxygen Supply

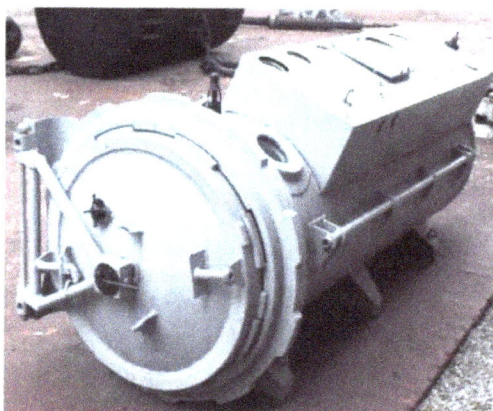

A recompression chamber for a single diving casualty

In the larger multiplace chambers, patients inside the chamber breathe from either "oxygen hoods" – flexible, transparent soft plastic hoods with a seal around the neck similar to a space suit helmet – or tightly fitting oxygen masks, which supply pure oxygen and may be designed to directly exhaust the exhaled gas from the chamber. During treatment patients breathe 100% oxygen most of the time to maximise the effectiveness of their treatment, but have periodic "air breaks" during which they breathe chamber air (21% oxygen) to reduce the risk of oxygen toxicity. The exhaled treatment gas must be removed from the chamber to prevent the buildup of oxygen, which could present a fire risk. Attendants may also breathe oxygen some of the time to reduce their risk of decompression sickness when they leave the chamber. The pressure inside the chamber is increased by opening valves allowing high-pressure air to enter from storage cylinders, which are filled by an air compressor. Chamber air oxygen content is kept between 19% and 23% to control fire risk (US Navy maximum 25%). If the chamber does not have a scrubber sysytem to remove carbon dioxide from the chamber gas, the chamber must be isobarically ventilated to keep the CO_2 within acceptable limits.

A soft chamber may be pressurised directly from a compressor. or from storage cylinders.

Smaller "monoplace" chambers can only accommodate the patient, and no medical staff can enter. The chamber may be pressurised with pure oxygen or compressed air. If pure oxygen is used, no oxygen breathing mask or helmet is needed, but the cost of using pure oxygen is much higher than that of using compressed air. If compressed air is used, then an oxygen mask or hood is needed as in a multiplace chamber. Most monoplace chambers can be fitted with a demand breathing system for air breaks. In low pressure soft chambers, treatment schedules may not require air breaks, because the risk of oxygen toxicity is low due to the lower oxygen partial pressures used (usually 1.3 ATA), and short duration of treatment.

For alert, cooperative patients, air breaks provided by mask are more effective than changing the chamber gas because they provide a quicker gas change and a more reliable gas composition both during the break and treatment periods.

Treatments

Initially, HBOT was developed as a treatment for diving disorders involving bubbles of gas in the tissues, such as decompression sickness and gas embolism, It is still considered the definitive treatment for these conditions. The chamber treats decompression sickness and gas embolism by increasing pressure, reducing the size of the gas bubbles and improving the transport of blood to downstream tissues. The high concentrations of oxygen in the tissues are beneficial in keeping oxygen-starved tissues alive, and have the effect of removing the nitrogen from the bubble, making it smaller until it consists only of oxygen, which is re-absorbed into the body. After elimination of bubbles, the pressure is gradually reduced back to atmospheric levels. Hyperbaric chambers are also used for animals, especially race horses where a recovery is worth a great deal to their owners. It is also used to treat dogs and cats in pre- and post-surgery treatment to strengthen their systems prior to surgery and then accelerate healing post surgery.

Protocol

The slang term, at some facilities, for a cycle of pressurization inside the HBOT chamber is "a dive". An HBOT treatment for longer-term conditions is often a series of 20 to 40 dives, or compressions. These dives last for about an hour and can be administered via a hard, high-pressure chamber or a soft, low-pressure chamber—the major difference being per-dive "dose" of oxygen. Many conditions do quite well with the lower dose, lower cost-per-hour, soft chambers.

Emergency HBOT for decompression illness follows treatment schedules laid out in treatment tables. Most cases employ a recompression to 2.8 bars (41 psi) absolute, the equivalent of 18 metres (60 ft) of water, for 4.5 to 5.5 hours with the casualty breathing pure oxygen, but taking air breaks every 20 minutes to reduce oxygen toxicity. For extremely serious cases resulting from very deep dives, the treatment may require a chamber capable of a maximum pressure of 8 bars (120 psi), the equivalent of 70 metres (230 ft) of water, and the ability to supply heliox as a breathing gas.

U.S. Navy treatment charts are used in Canada and the United States to determine the duration, pressure, and breathing gas of the therapy. The most frequently used tables are Table 5 and Table 6. In the UK the Royal Navy 62 and 67 tables are used.

The Undersea and Hyperbaric Medical Society (UHMS) publishes a report that compiles the latest research findings and contains information regarding the recommended duration and pressure of the longer-term conditions.

Home and Out-patient Clinic Treatment

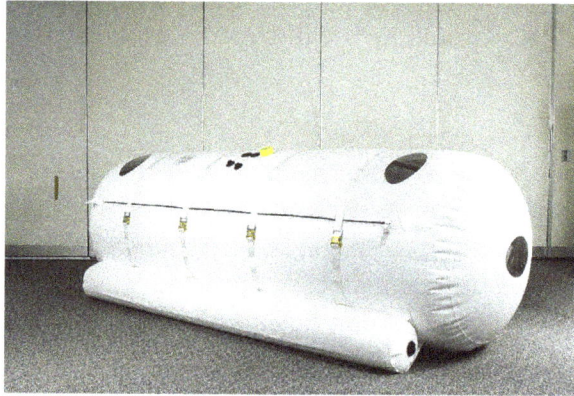

An example of mild portable hyperbaric chamber. This 40-inch-diameter (1,000 mm) chamber is one of the larger chambers available for home.

There are several sizes of portable chambers, which are used for home treatment. These are usually referred to as "mild personal hyperbaric chambers", which is a reference to the lower pressure (compared to hard chambers) of soft-sided chambers. Food and Drug Administration (FDA) approved chambers for use with room air are available in the USA and may go up to 4.4 pounds per square inch (psi) above atmospheric pressure, which equals 1.3 atmospheres absolute (ATA), equivalent to a depth of 10 feet of sea water. In the US, these "mild personal hyperbaric chambers" are categorized by the FDA as CLASS II medical devices and requires a prescription in order to purchase one or take treatments. Personal hyperbaric chambers are only FDA approved to reach 1.3 ATA. While hyperbaric chamber distributors and manufacturers cannot supply a chamber in the US with any form of elevated oxygen delivery system, a physician can write a prescription to combine the two modalities, as long as there is a prescription for both hyperbarics and oxygen. The most common option (but not approved by FDA) some patients choose is to acquire an oxygen concentrator which typically delivers 85–96% oxygen as the breathing gas. Because of the high circulation of air through the chamber, the total concentration of oxygen in the chamber never exceeds 25% as this can increase the risk of fire. Oxygen is never fed directly into soft chambers but is rather introduced via a line and mask directly to the patient. FDA approved oxygen concentrators for human consumption in confined areas used for HBOT are regularly monitored for purity (+/- 1%) and flow (10 to 15 liters per minute outflow pressure). An audible alarm will sound if the purity ever drops below 80%. Personal hyperbaric chambers use 120 volt or 220 volt outlets. Ranging in size from 21 inches up to 40 inches in diameter these chambers measure between 84 in (7 ft) to 120 in (10 ft) in length. The soft chambers are approved by the FDA for the treatment of altitude sickness, but are commonly used for other "off-label" purposes.

Possible Complications and Concerns

There are risks associated with HBOT, similar to some diving disorders. Pressure changes can cause a "squeeze" or barotrauma in the tissues surrounding trapped air inside the body, such as the lungs, behind the eardrum, inside paranasal sinuses, or trapped underneath dental fillings. Breathing high-pressure oxygen may cause oxygen toxicity. Temporarily blurred vision can be caused by swelling of the lens, which usually resolves in two to four weeks.

There are reports that cataract may progress following HBOT. Also a rare side effect has been blindness secondary to optic neuritis (inflammation of the optic nerve).

Effects of Pressure

Patients inside the chamber may notice discomfort inside their ears as a pressure difference develops between their middle ear and the chamber atmosphere. This can be relieved by ear clearing using the Valsalva maneuver or other techniques. Continued increase of pressure without equalising may cause ear drums to rupture, resulting in severe pain. As the pressure in the chamber increases further, the air may become warm.

To reduce the pressure, a valve is opened to allow air out of the chamber. As the pressure falls, the patient's ears may "squeak" as the pressure inside the ear equalizes with the chamber. The temperature in the chamber will fall. The speed of pressurization and de-pressurization can be adjusted to each patient's needs.

Costs

HBOT is recognized by Medicare in the United States as a reimbursable treatment for

14 UHMS "approved" conditions. A 1-hour HBOT session may cost between $165 and $250 in private clinics, and over $2,000 in hospitals. U.S. physicians (either M.D., D.O., D.D.S., D.M.D., D.C.) may lawfully prescribe HBOT for "off-label" conditions such as stroke, and migraine. Such patients are treated in outpatient clinics. In the United Kingdom most chambers are financed by the National Health Service, although some, such as those run by Multiple Sclerosis Therapy Centres, are non-profit. In Australia, HBOT is not covered by Medicare as a treatment for multiple sclerosis. The average U.S. hospital charge is $1,800.00 per 90 minute HBOT treatment. China and Russia treat more than 80 maladies, conditions and trauma with HBOT.

Research

The University of Birmingham's 2012 guidance to West Midlands primary care trusts and clinical commissioning groups concluded "The primary research studies investigating the efficacy of HBO are remarkable for the consistent poor quality of the published clinical trials as well as the lack of evidence demonstrating significant health benefits. There is a lack of adequate clinical evidence to support the view that HBO therapy is efficacious for any of the indications for which it is being used".

Aspects under research include radiation-induced hemorrhagic cystitis; and inflammatory bowel disease.

Neurological

Tentative evidence shows a possible benefit in cerebrovascular diseases. The clinical experience and results so far published has promoted the use of HBO therapy in patients with cerebrovascular injury and focal cerebrovascular injuries. However, the power of clinical research is limited because of the shortage of randomized controlled trials.

Radiation Wounds

A 2010 review of studies of HBOT applied to wounds from radiation therapy reported that, while most studies suggest a beneficial effect, more experimental and clinical research is needed to validate its clinical use.

History

Hyperbaric Air

The use of air at raised ambient pressure for the treatment of illness is recorded from 1662 for afflictions of the lung, by Henshaw. It is unlikely to have had any significant effect.

Junod built a chamber in France in 1834 to treat pulmonary conditions at pressures between 2 and 4 atmospheres absolute.

During the following century "pneumatic centres" were established in Europe and the USA which used hyperbaric air to treat a variety of conditions.

Orval J Cunningham, a professor of anaesthesia at the University of Kansas in the early 1900s observed that people suffering from circulatory disorders did better at sea level than at altitude and this formed the basis for his use of hyperbaric air. In 1918 he successfully treated patients suffering from the Spanish flu with hyperbaric air. In 1930 the American Medical Association forced him to stop hyperbaric treatment, since he did not provide acceptable evidence that the treatments were effective.

Hyperbaric Oxygen

The English scientist Joseph Priestley discovered oxygen in 1775. Shortly after its discovery, there were reports of toxic effects of hyperbaric oxygen on the central nervous system and lungs, which delayed therapeutic applications until 1937, when Behnke and Shaw first used it in the treatment of decompression sickness.

In 1955 and 1956 Churchill-Davidson, in the UK, used hyperbaric oxygen to enhance the radiosensitivity of tumours, while Ite Boerema, at the University of Amsterdam, successfully used it in cardiac surgery.

In 1961 WH Brummelkamp et al. published on the use of hyperbaric oxygen in the treatment of clostridial gas gangrene.

In 1962 Smith and Sharp reported successful treatment of carbon monoxide poisoning with hyperbaric oxygen.

The Undersea Medical Society (now Undersea and Hyperbaric Medical Society) formed a Committee on Hyperbaric Oxygenation which has become recognized as the authority on indications for hyperbaric oxygen treatment.

Wilderness Medicine (Practice)

Wilderness medicine, providing "vital emergency care in remote settings" is a rapidly evolving field and is of increasing importance as more people engage in hiking, climbing, kayaking and other potentially hazardous activities in the backcountry. A primary focus of the field is the evaluation, prioritization (triage), preliminary treatment of acute injuries or illnesses which occur in those environments and the emergency evacuation of victims. However, back country rescue and wilderness first aid is not the sole activity of wilderness medical professionals, who are also concerned with many additional topics. These include but are not limited to:

- secondary care follow up to first aid in remote settings, such as expeditions

- evaluation of experience and issuance of updated protocols for first response and secondary care

- the prevention of wilderness medical emergencies,

- epidemiological studies,

- public policy advisement to wilderness planning agencies, issuance of guidelines to disaster planning agencies, professional guides and amateur back country enthusiast organizations.

Scope of Wilderness Medicine

Wilderness medicine is a varied sub-speciality, encompassing skills and knowledge from many other specialties.

Diving and Hyperbaric Medicine

- Physics & Physiology of Depth

- Dive Medicine

- Dysbarisms & Barotrauma

Tropical and Travel Medicine

- Immunizations for Travel

- Tick-borne Illness, Malaria and Tropical Diseases

- Parasites & Protozoal infections in the Traveler

- Traveler's Diarrhea

- Women's Issues in Traveling

- Safety & Security While Traveling

- Travel Medicine

- Travel Dermatology

- Fever in the Returned Traveler & VHFs

- STDs in the Adventure Traveler

High-altitude and Mountaineering Medicine

- Physics & Physiology of Altitude

- AMS, HAPE & HACE

- The Effect of High Altitude on Underlying Medical Conditions

Expedition Medicine

- Basic Field Dentistry

- Expedition Planning, pre- and post- expedition responsibilities

Survival, Field Craft and Equipment

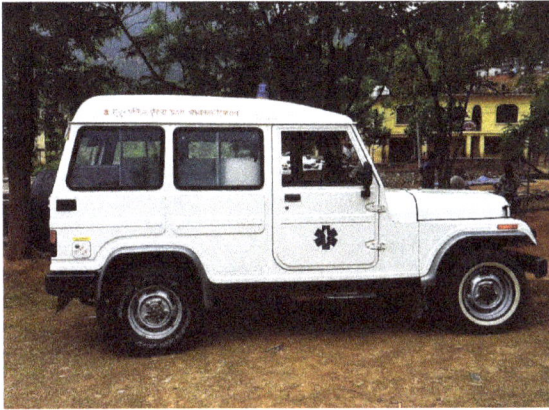

Casualty extrication by road

- Survival Techniques and equipment

- Water Procurement

- Food Procurement

- Hiking & Trekking

- Foot Gear and Care of the Feet & Clothing Selection for Wilderness Survival

- Land Navigation

Safety, Rescue and Evacuation

- Search and Rescue theory and practice

- Evacuation of Injured Persons

Sports Medicine and Physiology

Preventive Medicine, Field Sanitation and Hygiene

- Field Sanitation and Hygiene Measures

- Vector Control and Barriers

- Water Purification Methods

General Environmental Medicine

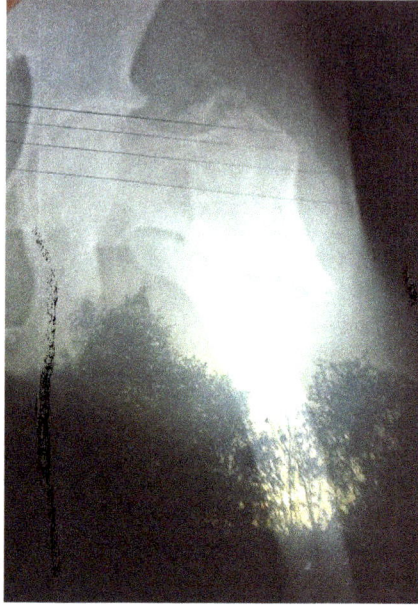

Using the sky as a lightbox

- Lightning Injuries

- Submersion and drowning

- Envenomation, Toxicology and Animal Attacks

- Heat Illness and Dehydration

- Cold injuries and Hypothermia

- Nutrition in Extreme Environments

- Aerospace Medicine

Improvised Medicine

- Improvised Field Wound Management

- Improvisational Medical Techniques in the Wilderness

Disaster and Humanitarian Assistance

- Triage

- Field Hospital provision

- Malnutrition therapy

Wilderness Emergencies and Trauma Management

- Pre-hospital Patient Assessment

- Pain Management in the Wilderness Setting

- Emergency Airway Management

- Psychological Response to Injury and Stress

- Management of Trauma and Injuries

Epidemiology

The Center for Disease Control in the U.S., as its corresponding agencies in other nations, also monitor pathogen vectors in conjunction with local departments of health, such as Lyme disease, plague and typhus which may be carried by small mammals in a back country or wilderness context.

Austere Environments Interdisciplinary Interface

Insights from the field of Military Combat Tactical Care (TCCC) interact with wilderness medical practice and protocol development. Moreover, new products and technologies tested in combat are adopted by wilderness medical personnel and vice versa.

References

- Stein, L (2000). "Dental Distress. The 'Diving Dentist' Addresses the Problem of a Diving-Related Toothache" (PDF). Alert Diver (January/ February): 45–48. Retrieved 2008-05-23

- Sakr, M (2000). "Casualty, accident and emergency, or emergency medicine, the evolution". Emergency Medicine Journal. 17 (5): 314–9. doi:10.1136/emj.17.5.314. PMC 1725462. PMID 11005398

- Emergency Medical Technician (EMT) (Speedy Study Guide). Speedy Publishing LLC. 2014. p. 1. ISBN 9781635011951

- Noyer CM, Brandt LJ (February 1999). "Hyperbaric oxygen therapy for perineal Crohn's disease". The American Journal of Gastroenterology. 94 (2): 318–321. doi:10.1111/j.1572-0241.1999.00848.x. PMID 10022622

- "Definition of Emergency Medicine". Clinical & Practice Management. American College of Emergency Physicians. Retrieved November 16, 2016

- Epstein, Arnold M. (2012). "Will Pay for Performance Improve Quality of Care? The Answer is in the Details". New England Journal of Medicine. 367 (19): 1852–3. doi:10.1056/NEJMe1212133. PMID 23134388

- Gesell, Laurie B. (2008). Hyperbaric Oxygen Therapy Indications. The Hyperbaric Oxygen

Therapy Committee Report (12th ed.). Durham, NC: Undersea and Hyperbaric Medical Society. ISBN 0-930406-23-0

- "A Matter of Urgency: Reducing Emergency Department Overuse" (PDF). NEHI Research Brief. New England Healthcare Institute. March 2010. Retrieved November 16, 2016

- Cho, E; Akkapeddi, V; Rajagopalan, A. "Developing Emerg Med Through Primary Care". National Medical Journal of India. 18 (3): 154–156

- Lampl LA, Frey G, Dietze T, Trauschel M (1989). "Hyperbaric Oxygen in Intracranial Abscesses". J. Hyperbaric Med. 4 (3): 111–126. Retrieved 2008-05-19

- Brubakk, A. O.; T. S. Neuman (2003). Bennett and Elliott's physiology and medicine of diving (5th Rev ed.). United States: Saunders Ltd. p. 800. ISBN 0-7020-2571-2

- Singhal AB, Lo EH (Feb 2008). "Advances in emerging nondrug therapies for acute stroke 2007". Stroke: A Journal of Cerebral Circulation. 39 (2): 289–291. doi:10.1161/STROKEAHA.107.511485. PMID 18187678

- "Characteristics of Frequent Emergency Department Users" (PDF). The Henry J. Kaiser Family Foundation. October 2007. Retrieved November 16, 2016

- Suter, Robert E (2012). "Emergency medicine in the United States: A systemic review". World Journal of Emergency Medicine. 3 (1): 5–10. doi:10.5847/wjem.j.issn.1920-8642.2012.01.001. PMC 4129827. PMID 25215031

- Marx, JA, ed. (2002). "chapter 194". Rosen's Emergency Medicine: Concepts and Clinical Practice (5th ed.). Mosby. ISBN 978-0323011853

- "42 U.S. Code § 1395dd - Examination and treatment for emergency medical conditions and women in labor". LII / Legal Information Institute. Retrieved 2016-11-19

- Hatley, T; Patterson, P. D. (2007). "Management and financing of emergency medical services". North Carolina medical journal. 68 (4): 259–61. PMID 17694845

- "$22.1 Million to Improve Access to Health Care in Rural Areas" (Press release). Health Resources and Services Administration. September 26, 2014. Retrieved January 29, 2017

- Marco, Catherine; et al. (2011). "Ethics Curriculum for Emergency Medicine Graduate Medical Education" (PDF). The Journal of Emergency Medicine Graduate Medical Education. 40: 5 – via Elsevier. CS1 maint: Explicit use of et al. (link)

- "When Doctors Admit Mistakes, Fewer Malpractice Suits Result, Study Says". Health News / Tips & Trends / Celebrity Health. 2010-08-17. Retrieved 2016-11-19

- Knight, John (June 2000). "Certification in diving and hyperbaric medicine in America and Australia". SPUMS Journal. South Pacific Underwater Medicine Society. 30 (2). Retrieved 2013-04-03

- "Emergency Medical Technicians and Paramedics". United States Department of Labor, Bureau of Labor Statistics. Retrieved 2008-03-10

Emergency Medical Equipment: An Overview

Spinal board is a device used to carry a patient with spinal or limb injuries. It is designed with the purpose of providing rigid support to the patient. The other medical equipment mentioned are automated external defibrillator, autopulse, cervical collar, splint, vacuum mattress, etc. This chapter is an overview of the subject matter incorporating all the major aspects of first aid and emergency medicine.

Spinal Board

A spinal board, is a patient handling device used primarily in pre-hospital trauma care.

It is designed to provide rigid support during movement of a person with suspected spinal or limb injuries. They are most commonly used by ambulance staff, as well as lifeguards and ski patrollers. Historically, backboards were also used in an attempt to "improve the posture" of young people, especially girls.

Due to lack of evidence to support long-term use, the practice of keeping people on long boards for prolonged periods of time is decreasing.

Extraction Uses

The spinal backboard was originally designed as a device to remove people from a vehicle. After a time people were simply kept on the spine board for transport without evidence supporting this need.

Medical Uses

A spinal board is primarily indicated for judicious use to transport people who may have had a spinal injury, usually due to the mechanism of injury, and the attending team are not able to rule out a spinal injury. The person should be transferred from the board to a hospital bed as soon as possible. For comfort and safety reasons, it is recommended to transfer the patient to a vacuum mattress instead, in which case a scoop stretcher or long spine board is just used for the transfer.

Despite its history of use, there is no evidence that backboards significantly immobilize the spine, nor do they improve patient outcomes. Additionally, cervical spine immobilization has been shown to increase mortality in patients with penetrating trauma and can cause pain, agitation, respiratory compromise, and can lead to the development of bedsores.

Adverse Effects

Common clinical issues found with spinal boards include pressure sore development, inadequacy of spinal immobilization, pain and discomfort, respiratory compromise and effects on the quality of radiological imaging. For this reason, some professionals view them as unsuitable for the task, preferring alternatives.

It is advised that no patient should spend more than 30 minutes on a spine board, due to the development of discomfort and pressure sores.

Backboards were invented to be a "highly polished surface" to move a person to an EMS bed, not to be used as spinal securing device.

Construction

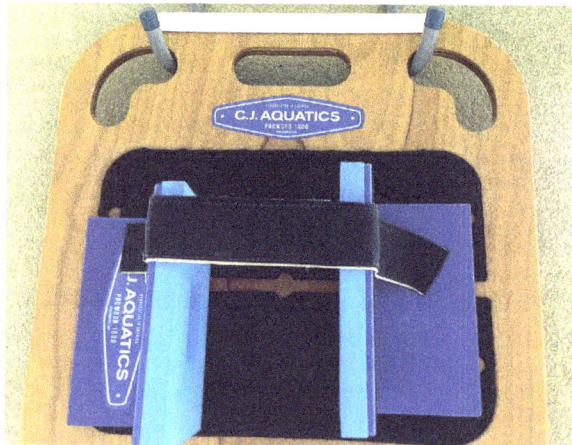

Head immobilizer at the top of the backboard.

Backboards are almost always used in conjunction with the following devices:

- a cervical collar with occipital padding as needed;

- side head supports, such as a rolled blanket or head blocks (head immobilizer) made specifically for this purpose, used to avoid the lateral rotation of the head;

- straps to secure the patient to the long spine board, and tape to secure the head

Spine boards are typically made of wood or plastic, although there has been a strong shift away from wood boards due to their higher level of maintenance required to keep them in operable condition and to protect them from cracks and other imperfections that could harbor bacteria.

Backboards are designed to be slightly wider and longer than the average human body to accommodate the immobilization straps, and have handles for carrying the patient. Most backboards are designed to be completely X-ray translucent so that they do not interfere with the exam while patients are strapped to them. They are light enough to be easily carried by one person, and are usually buoyant.

Alternatives

The vacuum mattress may reduce sacral pressures compared to backboards. The conforming nature of the vacuum mattress means that patients can be kept immobilized on it for longer periods of time and the immobilisation offers superior stability and comfort to the patient. The Kendrick extrication device is another alternative.

Automated External Defibrillator

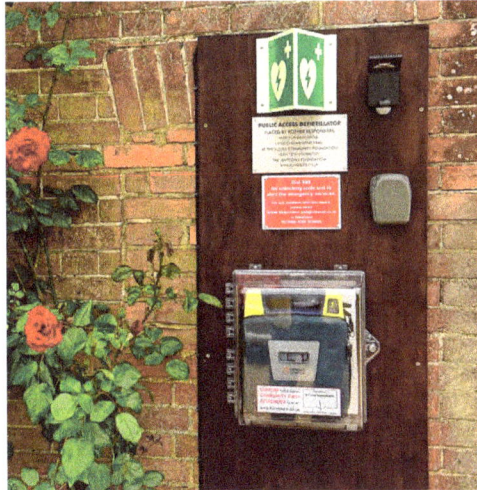

An automated external defibrillator (AED) ready for use. Pads are pre-connected. This model is a semi-automatic due to the presence of a shock button, Fully-automatic model also available by Cardiac Science.

An automated external defibrillator (AED) is a portable electronic device that automatically diagnoses the life-threatening cardiac arrhythmias of ventricular fibrillation and pulseless ventricular tachycardia in a patient, and is able to treat them through defibrillation, the application of electrical therapy which stops the arrhythmia, allowing the heart to reestablish an effective rhythm.

With simple audio and visual commands, AEDs are designed to be simple to use for the layperson, and the use of AEDs is taught in many first aid, certified first responder, and basic life support (BLS) level cardiopulmonary resuscitation (CPR) classes.

The portable version of the defibrillator was invented in the mid-1960s by Frank Pantridge in Belfast, Northern Ireland, a pioneer in emergency medical treatment.

Indications

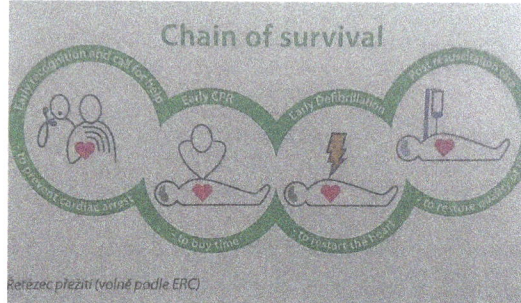

Chain of survival - every minute counts. AEDs save lives.

Conditions that the Device Treats

An automated external defibrillator is used in cases of life-threatening cardiac arrhythmias which lead to cardiac arrest. The rhythms that the device will treat are usually limited to:

1. Pulseless Ventricular tachycardia (shortened to VT or V-Tach)

2. Ventricular fibrillation (shortened to VF or V-Fib)

In each of these two types of shockable cardiac arrhythmia, the heart is electrically active, but in a dysfunctional pattern that does not allow it to pump and circulate blood. In ventricular tachycardia, the heart beats too fast to effectively pump blood. Ultimately, ventricular tachycardia leads to ventricular fibrillation. In ventricular fibrillation, the electrical activity of the heart becomes chaotic, preventing the ventricle from effectively pumping blood. The fibrillation in the heart decreases over time, and will eventually reach asystole.

AEDs, like all defibrillators, are not designed to shock asystole ('flat line' patterns) as this will not have a positive clinical outcome. The asystolic patient only has a chance of survival if, through a combination of CPR and cardiac stimulant drugs, one of the shockable rhythms can be established, which makes it imperative for CPR to be carried out prior to the arrival of a defibrillator.

Effect of Delayed Treatment

Uncorrected, these cardiac conditions (ventricular tachycardia, ventricular fibrillation, asystole) rapidly lead to irreversible brain damage and death, once cardiac arrest takes place. After approximately three to five minutes in cardiac arrest, irreversible brain/tissue damage may begin to occur. For every minute that a person in cardiac arrest goes without being successfully treated (by defibrillation), the chance of survival decreases by 7 percent per minute in the first 3 minutes, and decreases by 10 percent per minute as time advances beyond ~3 minutes.

Requirements for Use

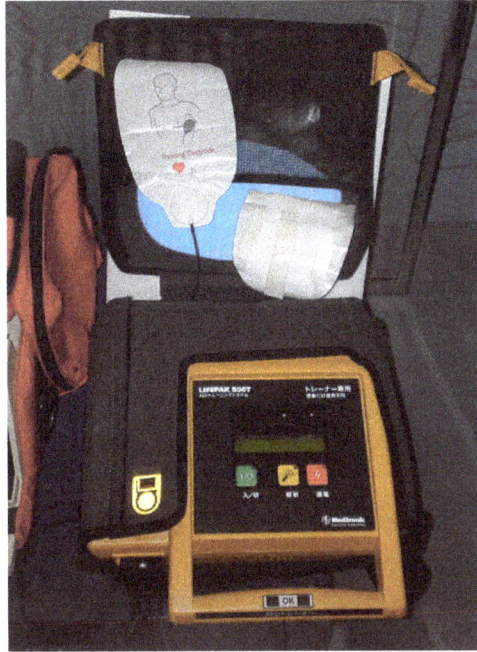

Defibrillator training kit

AEDs are designed to be used by laypersons who ideally should have received AED training. However, sixth-grade students have been reported to begin defibrillation within 90 seconds, as opposed to a trained operator beginning within 67 seconds. This is in contrast to more sophisticated manual and semi-automatic defibrillators used by health professionals, which can act as a pacemaker if the heart rate is too slow (bradycardia) and perform other functions which require a skilled operator able to read electrocardiograms.

Bras with a metal underwire and piercings on the torso must be removed before using the AED on someone to avoid interference. American TV show Mythbusters found evidence that use of a defibrillator on a woman wearing an underwire bra can lead to arcing or fire but only in unusual and unlikely circumstances.

A study analyzed the effects of having AEDs immediately present during Chicago's Heart Start program over a two-year period. Of 22 individuals 18 were in a cardiac arrhythmia which AEDs can treat (Vfib or Vtach). Of these 18, 11 survived. Of these 11 patients, 6 were treated by bystanders with absolutely no previous training in AED use.

Implementation

Placement and Availability

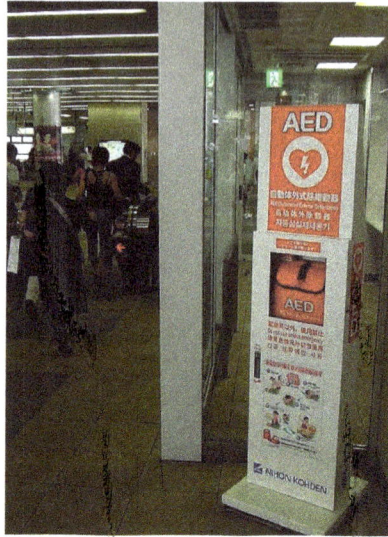

An AED at a railway station in Japan.

Automated external defibrillators are generally either kept with trained personnel who will attend events or are public access units which can be found in places including corporate and government offices, shopping centres, airports, airplanes, restaurants, casinos, hotels, sports stadiums, schools and universities, community centers, fitness centers, health clubs, theme parks, workplaces and any other location where people may congregate.

The location of a public access AED should take into account where large groups of people gather, regardless of age or activity. Children as well as adults may fall victim to sudden cardiac arrest (SCA).

In many areas, emergency vehicles are likely to carry AEDs, with some ambulances carrying an AED in addition to manual defibrillators. Police or fire vehicles often carry an AED for use by first responders. Some areas have dedicated community first responders, who are volunteers tasked with keeping an AED and taking it to any victims in their area. AEDs are also increasingly common on commercial airliners, cruise ships, and other transportation facilities.

High-rise buildings are densely populated, but are more difficult to access by emergency crews facing heavy traffic and security barriers. It has been suggested that AEDs carried on elevators could save critical minutes for cardiac arrest victims, and reduce their deployment cost.

In order to make them highly visible, public access AEDs are often brightly colored, and are mounted in protective cases near the entrance of a building. When these protective cases are opened or the defibrillator is removed, some will sound a buzzer to alert near-by staff to their removal, though this does not necessarily summon emergency services; trained AED operators should know to phone for an ambulance when sending for or using an AED. In September 2008, the International Liaison Committee on Resuscitation issued a 'universal AED sign' to be adopted throughout the world to indicate the presence of an AED.

A trend that is developing is the purchase of AEDs to be used in the home, particularly by those with known existing heart conditions. The number of devices in the community has grown as prices have fallen to affordable levels. There has been some concern among medical professionals that these home users do not necessarily have appropriate training, and many advocate the more widespread use of community responders, who can be appropriately trained and managed.

Typically, an AED kit will contain a face shield for providing a barrier between patient and first aider during rescue breathing; a pair of nitrile rubber gloves; a pair of trauma shears for cutting through a patient's clothing to expose the chest; a small towel for wiping away any moisture on the chest, and a razor for shaving those with very hairy chests.

Preparation for Operation

Most manufacturers recommend checking the AED before every period of duty or on a regular basis for fixed units. Some units need to be switched on in order to perform a self check; other models have a self check system built in with a visible indicator.

All manufacturers mark their electrode pads with an expiration date, and it is important to ensure that the pads are in date. This is usually marked on the outside of the pads. Some models are designed to make this date visible through a 'window', although others will require the opening of the case to find the date stamp.

It is also important to ensure that the AED unit's batteries have not expired. The AED manufacturer will specify how often the batteries should be replaced. Each AED has a different recommended maintenance schedule outlined in the user manual. Common checkpoints on every checklist, however, also include a monthly check of the battery power by checking the green indicator light when powered on, condition and cleanliness of all cables and the unit, and check for the adequate supplies

To ensure that AED is working properly at all times, the D-Box telemetry device can be used. It connects to an AED device, recognizes the particular device's beeps and knows that it beeps in just this particular way when it's broken. In a situation when an AED has stopped working, the D-Box sends notifications and lets you discover problems before it's too late.

Mechanism of Operation

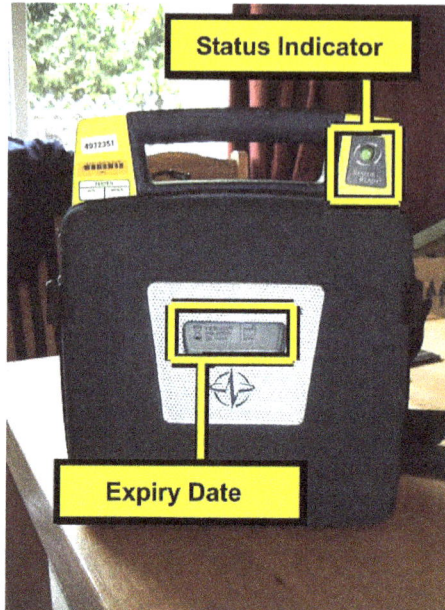

The use of easily visible status indicator and pad expiration date on a Cardiac Science G3 AED

An AED is "automatic" because of the unit's ability to autonomously analyse the patient's condition. To assist this, the vast majority of units have spoken prompts, and some may also have visual displays to instruct the user.

"External" refers to the fact that the operator applies the electrode pads to the bare chest of the victim (as opposed to internal defibrillators, which have electrodes surgically implanted inside the body of a patient).

When turned on or opened, the AED will instruct the user to connect the electrodes (pads) to the patient. Once the pads are attached, everyone should avoid touching the patient so as to avoid false readings by the unit. The pads allow the AED to examine the electrical output from the heart and determine if the patient is in a shockable rhythm (either ventricular fibrillation or ventricular tachycardia). If the device determines that a shock is warranted, it will use the battery to charge its internal capacitor in preparation to deliver the shock. This system is not only safer (charging only when required), but also allows for a faster delivery of the electric current.

When charged, the device instructs the user to ensure no one is touching the patient and then to press a button to deliver the shock; human intervention is usually required to deliver the shock to the patient in order to avoid the possibility of accidental injury to another person (which can result from a responder or bystander touching the patient at the time of the shock). Depending on the manufacturer and particular model, after the shock is delivered most devices will analyze the patient and either instruct CPR to be given, or administer another shock.

Many AED units have an 'event memory' which store the ECG of the patient along with details of the time the unit was activated and the number and strength of any shocks delivered. Some units also have voice recording abilities to monitor the actions taken by the personnel in order to ascertain if these had any impact on the survival outcome. All this recorded data can be either downloaded to a computer or printed out so that the providing organisation or responsible body is able to see the effectiveness of both CPR and defibrillation. Some AED units even provide feedback on the quality of the compressions provided by the rescuer.

The first commercially available AEDs were all of a monophasic type, which gave a high-energy shock, up to 360 to 400 joules depending on the model. This caused increased cardiac injury and in some cases second and third-degree burns around the shock pad sites. Newer AEDs (manufactured after late 2003) have tended to utilise biphasic algorithms which give two sequential lower-energy shocks of 120 - 200 joules, with each shock moving in an opposite polarity between the pads. This lower-energy waveform has proven more effective in clinical tests, as well as offering a reduced rate of complications and reduced recovery time.

Geolocation

A standard logo is clearly advertised. The location is indicated in OpenStreetMap by the *emergency=defibrillator* tag.

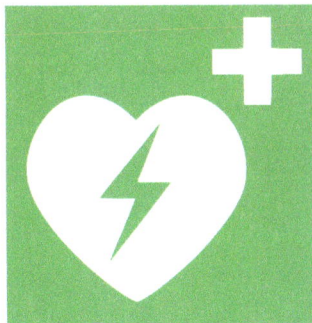

Usage

Simplicity of use

Unlike regular defibrillators, an automated external defibrillator requires minimal training to use. It automatically diagnoses the heart rhythm and determines if a shock is needed. Automatic models will administer the shock without the user's command. Semi-automatic models will tell the user that a shock is needed, but the user must tell the machine to do so, usually by pressing a button. In most circumstances, the user cannot override a "no shock" advisory by an AED. Some AEDs may be used on children - those under 55 lbs (25 kg) in weight or under age 8. If a particular model of AED is approved for pediatric use, all that is required is the use of more appropriate pads.

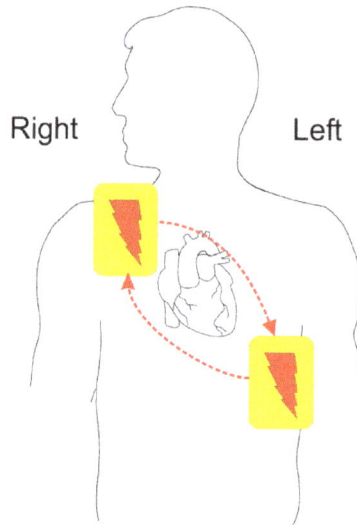

Usual placement of pads on chest

All AEDs approved for use in the United States use an electronic voice to prompt users through each step. Because the user of an AED may be hearing impaired, many AEDs now include visual prompts as well. Most units are designed for use by non-medical operators. Their ease of use has given rise to the notion of public access defibrillation (PAD), which experts agree has the potential to be the single greatest advance in the treatment of out-of-hospital cardiac arrest since the invention of CPR. Some advances include a CPR feedback device by Zoll and Cardiac Science, non-polarized pads (they can be placed in either location) by Cardiac Science, a status indicator most AEDS, and simple voice and text prompts with an adjustable skill level, on most AEDs.

Liability

Automated external defibrillators are now easy enough to use that most states in the United States include the "good faith" use of an AED by any person under Good Samaritan laws. "Good faith" protection under a Good Samaritan law means that a volunteer responder (not acting as a part of one's occupation) cannot be held civilly liable for the harm or death of a victim by providing improper or inadequate care, given that the harm or death was not intentional and the responder was acting within the limits of their training and in good faith. In the United States, Good Samaritan laws provide some protection for the use of AEDs by trained and untrained responders. AEDs create little liability if used correctly; NREMT-B and many state Emergency Medical Technician (EMT) training and many CPR classes incorporate or offer AED education as a part of their program. In addition to Good Samaritan laws, Ontario, Canada also has the "Chase McEachern Act (Heart Defibrillator Civil Liability), 2007 (Bill 171 – Subsection N)", passed in June, 2007, which protects individuals from liability for damages that may occur from their use of an AED to save someone's life at the immediate scene of an emergency unless damages are caused by gross negligence.

Reliability

Automated external defibrillators are under recent scrutiny by the U.S. Food and Drug Administration (FDA) which is now considering reclassifying AEDs as class III pre-market approval devices. The major reason for this appears to be technical malfunctions, which likely contributed to more than 750 deaths in the 5-year period between 2004 and 2009, in most cases by component failures or design errors. During the same period, up to 70 types of AEDs have been recalled, including recalls from every AED manufacturer in the world.

History

The first use of an external defibrillator on a human was in 1947 by Claude Beck. The portable version of the defibrillator was invented in the mid-1960s by Frank Pantridge in Belfast, Northern Ireland, a pioneer in emergency medical treatment.

AutoPulse

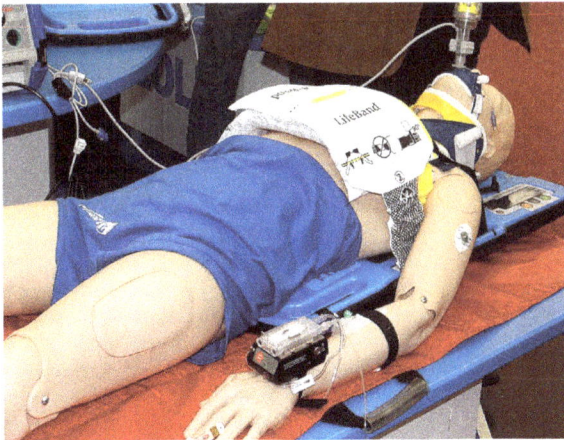
AutoPulse on a Dummy

The AutoPulse is an automated, portable, battery-powered cardiopulmonary resuscitation device created by Revivant and subsequently purchased and currently manufactured by ZOLL Medical Corporation. It is a chest compression device composed of a constricting band and half backboard that is intended to be used as an adjunct to CPR during advanced cardiac life support by professional health care providers. The Auto-Pulse uses a distributing band to deliver the chest compressions. In literature it is also known as LDB-CPR (Load Distributing Band-CPR).

The AutoPulse measures chest size and resistance before it delivers the unique combination of thoracic and cardiac chest compressions. The compression depth and force varies per patient. The chest displacement equals a 20% reduction in the anterior-posterior chest depth. The physiological duty cycle is 50%, and it runs in a 30:2, 15:2 or continuous compression mode, which is user-selectable, at a rate of 80 compressions-per-minute.

Device Operation

The patient's head, shoulders and upper back lay upon the base unit, with the controls for the AutoPulse beside the patient's left ear. It can be augmented for cervical spinal support. The unit contains the control computer, the rechargeable battery, and the motors that operate the LifeBand. The LifeBand is an adjustable strap that covers the entire rib cage. When the patient is strapped in and the start button is pressed, the LifeBand pulls tight around the chest, determines the patient's chest size and resistance, and proceeds to rhythmically constrict the entire rib cage, pumping the heart at a rate of 80 compressions per minute. The LifeBand can be placed over defibrillation pads. The LifeBand is disposable, and designed to be used on a single patient for sanitary reasons.

Mechanism of CPR Blood Flow

The load-distributing band system, employing thoracic compressions, produces higher blood flow compared to CPR consisting of sternal compressions only. The potential to produce blood flow for a sudden cardiac arrest victim is in large part determined by the peak power of the compression. Factors determining the power of the compression are the force of the compression, the depth of the compression, and the duration that the compression is held at maximum depth.

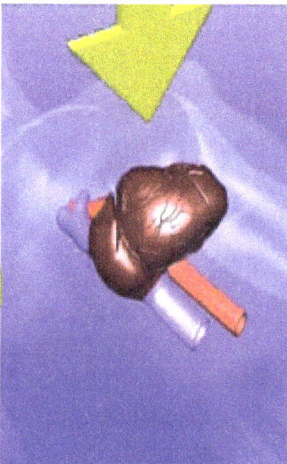

Thoracic and Cardiac Pump combined

Cardiac Pump - Compresses mainly the heart

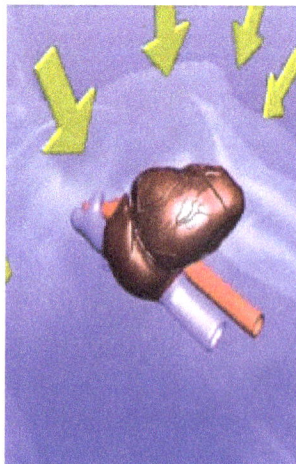

Thoracic Pump - Compresses the entire chest

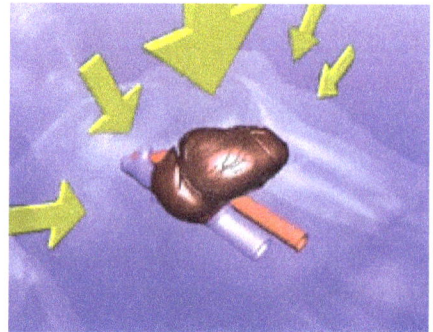

Studies and clinical trials

The gold standard for resuscitation research is *survival to hospital discharge*. Although common sense suggests that short-term and intermediate outcomes like *return of spontaneous circulation (ROSC)* or *survival to hospital admission* are promising, experienced scientists know that anything less than a neurologically intact survivor walking out of the hospital is ultimately irrelevant.

Several animal studies have shown that automated CPR machines are more effective at providing circulatory support than manual CPR. One study showed that use of the AutoPulse produced blood flow to the heart and brain that was comparable to pre-arrest levels. In another study, an adapted AutoPulse was shown to be highly effective in support of cardiac arrest in animals, whereas manual CPR was tenuous in its effectiveness. Pigs were used in the study, and were left in cardiac arrest for eight minutes to simulate average ambulance response time. 73% of the pigs that were put into the AutoPulse were revived, and 88% of the surviving pigs showed no neurological damage. None of the pigs that received manual CPR survived.

The Circulation Improving Resuscitation Care (CIRC) trial is the largest prospective randomized trial to date for mechanical chest compressions in out-of-hospital cardiac arrest (OHCA). The goal was to demonstrate that the AutoPulse Non-invasive Cardiac Support Pump is a safe and effective component of a system of care focusing on high-quality chest compressions.

Compared to high-quality manual CPR, AutoPulse CPR resulted in statistically equivalent survival to hospital discharge and no difference in neurologic status at discharge in adults with out-of-hospital cardiac arrest of presumed cardiac etiology.

There are times when delivering high quality manual CPR isn't practical or even possible; the results of the CIRC trial confirm the important role the AutoPulse system can play in improving resuscitation outcomes.

The American Heart Association Guidelines for Cardiopulmonary Resuscitation give load-distributing band CPR (LDB-CPR) a Class IIb recommendation.

Class I	Definitely recommended. Supported by excellent evidence.
Class IIa	Acceptable and useful. Good to very good evidence provides support.
Class IIb	Acceptable and useful. Fair to good evidence provides support.
Class III	Unacceptable, no documented benefit, may be harmful.

In the News

Mirror, a U.K. news website, on January 14, 2011, reports on Arun Bhasin, who 'came back from the dead' after 3 and a half hours. He was found unconscious and brought into Croydon University Hospital. He suffered a cardiac arrest and was placed on the AutoPulse, which performed almost 20,000 compressions, keeping his heart and lungs functioning while a medical team worked on him. After almost 3 and a half hours, his pulse returned.

CNN's Anderson Cooper 360° featured a story on April 6, 2010, about the Firehouse Subs Public Safety Foundation, in which Firehouse Subs founders Chris and Robin Sorensen met with Francisco Tuttle, a father who was saved by the Mt. Pleasant, SC, Fire Department using a ZOLL AutoPulse, which the Foundation donated to the department last year.

ABC World News Tonight on September 22, 2004, did a story on automated CPR machines, and profiled the story of Caralee Weich, who survived thirty-five minutes of cardiac arrest during which the AutoPulse was used. She had a Sudden Cardiac Arrest in front of a theatre. Two nurses began immediate CPR. After a half-hour with no heartbeat, she ultimately recovered with no apparent brain damage.*MEDICINE ON THE CUTTING EDGE BETTER CPR (tape). ABC News. 2004.*

Criticism

The AutoPulse has received a fair amount of criticism surrounding its battery life, bulk, and studies suggesting poor survival to hospital discharge. The most notable case of such issues can be found in the news reports of the resuscitation of Prince Friso after he and his companion were caught in an avalanche. In that case, the AutoPulse batteries failed after only 9 and 15 minutes. Others have criticized the high cost and non-reimbursable nature of the disposable AutoPulse LifeBand.

The new AutoPulse Power System is based on intelligent technology that is designed to simplify maintenance of AutoPulse batteries by automating monthly conditioning. The AutoPulse can be operated with Li-Ion (lithium-ion) batteries which are designed for busy, mobile environments where weight is an overriding concern.

Studies have also failed to show an increase in survival to hospital discharge. During the ASPIRE trial (the first multi-centered, randomized trial with large enrollment), the survival to hospital discharge rates decreased from 9.9% with manual CPR to approximately 5%. Because of these findings, the ethics review board terminated the study. However, some researchers question the validity of the ASPIRE protocol. The CIRC study results additionally indicate that the AutoPulse increases the time before first defibrillation and decrease the average compressions per minute in comparison with manual CPR. Overall, the study shows no improvement over high quality manual CPR.

Several cases have been reported where the AutoPulse has caused additional injury to patients receiving compressions from the device.

Some departments and agencies have begun discontinuing the use of the AutoPulse, citing battery and reliability issues.

Bag Valve Mask

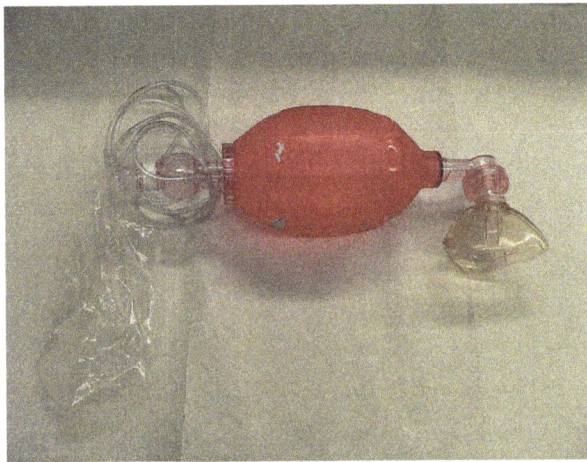

A disposable BVM Resuscitator

A bag valve mask, abbreviated to BVM and sometimes known by the proprietary name Ambu bag or generically as a manual resuscitator or "self-inflating bag", is a hand-held device commonly used to provide positive pressure ventilation to patients who are not breathing or not breathing adequately. The device is a required part of resuscitation kits for trained professionals in out-of-hospital settings (such as ambulance crews) and is also frequently used in hospitals as part of standard equipment found on a crash cart, in emergency rooms or other critical care settings. Underscoring the frequency and prominence of BVM use in the United States, the American Heart Association (AHA) Guidelines for Cardiopulmonary Resuscitation and Emergency Cardiac Care recommend that "all healthcare providers should be familiar with the use of the bag-mask device." Manual resuscitators are also used within the hospital for temporary ventilation of patients dependent on mechanical ventilators when the mechanical ventilator needs to be examined for possible malfunction, or when ventilator-dependent patients are transported within the hospital. Two principal types of manual resuscitators exist; one version is self-filling with air, although additional oxygen (O_2) can be added but is not necessary for the device to function. The other principal type of manual resuscitator (flow-inflation) is heavily used in non-emergency applications in the operating room to ventilate patients during anesthesia induction and recovery.

Use of manual resuscitators to ventilate a patient is frequently called "bagging" the patient and is regularly necessary in medical emergencies when the patient's breathing is insufficient (respiratory failure) or has ceased completely (respiratory arrest). Use of the manual resuscitator force-feeds air or oxygen into the lungs in order to inflate them under pressure, thus constituting a means to manually provide positive-pressure ventilation. It is used by professional rescuers in preference to mouth-to-mouth ventilation, either directly or through an adjunct such as a pocket mask.

History

The bag-valve mask concept was developed in 1953 by the German engineer Holger Hesse and his partner, Danish anaesthetist Henning Ruben, following their initial work on a suction pump. Later Hesse's company was renamed to Ambu, which has manufactured and market the device since the late 1950s. The full-form of AMBU is Artificial Manual Breathing Unit. An Ambu® bag is a self-inflating bag resuscitator from the company Ambu, who still manufactures and markets self-inflating bag resuscitators. Today there are several manufacturers of self-inflating bag resuscitators.

Standard Components

Mask

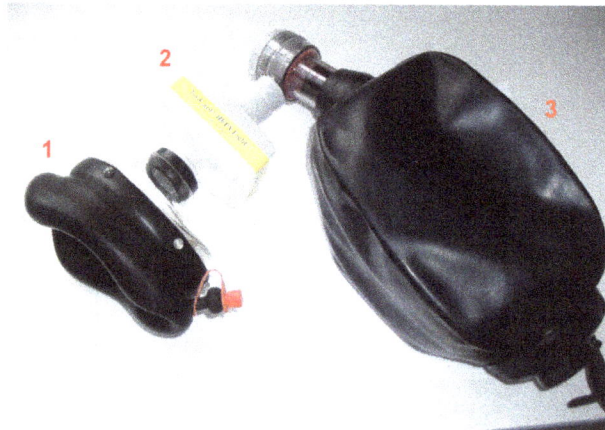

Bag valve mask. Part 1 is the flexible mask to seal over the patients face, part 2 has a filter and valve to prevent backflow into the bag itself (prevents patient deprivation and bag contamination) and part 3 is the soft bag element which is squeezed to expel air to the patient

The BVM consists of a flexible air chamber (the "bag", about the size of an American football), attached to a face mask via a shutter valve. When the face mask is properly applied and the "bag" is squeezed, the device forces air through into the patient's lungs; when the bag is released, it self-inflates from its other end, drawing in either ambient air or a low pressure oxygen flow supplied by a regulated cylinder, while also allowing the patient's lungs to deflate to the ambient environment (not the bag) past the one way valve.

Bag and Valve

Bag and valve combinations can also be attached to an alternate airway adjunct, instead of to the mask. For example, it can be attached to an endotracheal tube or laryngeal mask airway. Small heat and moisture exchangers, or humidifying / bacterial filters, can be used.

A bag-valve mask can be used without being attached to an oxygen tank to provide "room air" (21% oxygen) to the patient, however manual resuscitator devices also can be connected to a separate bag reservoir which can be filled with pure oxygen from a compressed oxygen source – this can increase the amount of oxygen delivered to the patient to nearly 100%.

Bag-valve masks come in different sizes to fit infants, children, and adults. The face mask size may be independent of the bag size; for example, a single pediatric-sized bag might be used with different masks for multiple face sizes, or a pediatric mask might be used with an adult bag for patients with small faces.

Most types of the device are disposable and therefore single use, while others are designed to be cleaned and reused.

Method of Operation

Manual resuscitators cause the gas inside the inflatable bag portion to be force-fed to the patient via a one-way valve when compressed by the rescuer; the gas is then ideally delivered through a mask and into the patient's trachea, bronchus and into the lungs. In order to be effective, a bag valve mask must deliver between 500 and 800 milliliters of air to a normal male adult patient's lungs, but if supplemental oxygen is provided 400 ml may still be adequate. Squeezing the bag once every 5 to 6 seconds for an adult or once every 3 seconds for an infant or child provides an adequate respiratory rate (10–12 respirations per minute in an adult and 20 per minute in a child or infant).

Professional rescuers are taught to ensure that the mask portion of the BVM is properly sealed around the patient's face (that is, to ensure proper "mask seal"); otherwise, pressure needed to force-inflate the lungs is released to the environment. This is difficult when a single rescuer attempts to maintain a face mask seal with one hand while squeezing the bag with other. Therefore, common protocol uses two rescuers: one rescuer to hold the mask to the patient's face with both hands and focus entirely on maintaining a leak-proof mask seal, while the other rescuer squeezes the bag and focuses on breath (or tidal volume) and timing.

An endotracheal tube (ET) can be inserted by an advanced practitioner and can substitute for the mask portion of the manual resuscitator. This provides more secure air passage between the resuscitator and the patient, since the ET tube is sealed with an inflatable cuff within the trachea (or windpipe), so any regurgitation is less likely to enter the lungs, and so that forced inflation pressure can only go into the lungs and not inadvertently go to the stomach. The ET tube also maintains an open and secure airway at all times, even during CPR compressions; as opposed to when a manual resuscitator is used with a mask when a face mask seal can be difficult to maintain during compressions.

Complications

Under normal breathing, the lungs inflate under a slight vacuum when the chest wall muscles and diaphragm expand; this "pulls" the lungs open, causing air to enter the lungs to inflate under a gentle vacuum. However, when using a manual resuscitator, as with other methods of positive-pressure ventilation, the lungs are force-inflated with pressurized air or oxygen. This inherently leads to risk of various complications, many of which depend on whether the manual resuscitator is being used with a face mask or ET tube. Complications are related to over-inflating or over-pressurizing the patient, which can cause: (1) air to inflate the stomach (called gastric insufflation); (2) lung injury from over-stretching (called volutrauma); and/or (3) lung injury from over-pressurization (called barotrauma).

Stomach Inflation / Lung Aspiration

When a face mask is used in conjunction with a manual resuscitator, the intent is for the force-delivered air or oxygen to inflate the lungs. However air entering the patient also has access to the stomach via the esophagus, which can inflate if the resuscitator is squeezed too hard (causing air flow that is too rapid for the lungs to absorb alone) or too much (causing excess air to divert to the stomach)." Gastric inflation can lead to vomiting and subsequent aspiration of stomach contents into the lungs, which has been cited as a major hazard of bag-valve-mask ventilation, with one study suggesting this effect is difficult to avoid even for the most skilled and experienced users, stating "When using a self-inflatable bag, even experienced anesthesiologists in our study may have performed ventilation with too short inspiratory times and/or too large tidal volumes, which resulted in stomach inflation in some cases." The study goes on to state that "Stomach inflation is a complex problem that may cause regurgitation, [gastric acid] aspiration, and, possibly, death." When stomach inflation leads to vomiting of highly acidic stomach acids, delivery of subsequent breaths can force these caustic acids down into the lungs where they cause life-threatening or fatal lung injuries including Mendelson's syndrome, aspiration pneumonia, adult respiratory distress syndrome and "pulmonary injuries similar to that seen in victims of chlorine gas exposure". Apart from the risks of gastric inflation causing vomiting and regurgitation, at least two reports have been found indicating that gastric insufflation itself remains clinically problematic even when vomiting does not occur. In one case of failed resuscitation (leading to death), gastric insufflation in a 3-month-old boy put sufficient pressure against the lungs that "precluded effective ventilation". Another reported complication was a case of stomach rupture caused by stomach over-inflation from a manual resuscitator. The causative factors and degree of risk of inadvertent stomach inflation have been examined, with one published study revealing that during prolonged resuscitation up to 75% of air delivered to the patient may inadvertently be delivered to the stomach instead of the lungs.

Lung Injury and Air Embolism

When an endotracheal (ET) tube is placed, one of the key advantages is that a direct airtight passageway is provided from the output of the manual resuscitator to the lungs, thus eliminating the possibilities of inadvertent stomach inflation or lung injuries from gastric acid aspiration. However this places the lungs at increased risk from separate lung injury patterns caused by accidental forced over-inflation (called volutrauma and/ or barotrauma). Sponge-like lung tissue is delicate, and over-stretching can lead to adult respiratory distress syndrome – a condition that requires prolonged mechanical ventilator support in the ICU and is associated with poor survival (e.g., 50%), and significantly increased care costs of up to $30,000 per day. Lung volutrauma, which can still be achieved through "careful" delivery of large, slow breaths, can also lead to a "popped" or collapsed lung (called a pneumothorax), with at least one published report describing "a patient in whom a sudden tension pneumothorax developed during ventilation with a bag-valve device." Additionally, there is at least one report of manual resuscitator use where the lungs were accidentally over-inflated to the point where "the heart contained a large volume of air," and the "aorta and pulmonary arteries were filled with air" – a condition called an air embolism which "is almost uniformly fatal".

Public Health Risk from Manual Resuscitator Complications

Two factors appear to make the public particularly at risk from complications from manual resuscitators: (1) their prevalence of use (leading to high probability of exposure), and (2) apparent inability for providers to protect patients from uncontrolled, inadvertent, forced over-inflation.

Prevalence of Manual Resuscitator use

Manual resuscitators are commonly used for temporary ventilation support, especially flow-inflation versions that are used during anesthesia induction/recovery during routine surgery. Accordingly, most citizens are likely to be "bagged" at least once during their lifetime as they undergo procedures involving general anesthesia. Additionally, a significant number of newborns are ventilated with infant-sized manual resuscitators to help stimulate normal breathing, making manual resuscitators among the very first therapeutic medical devices encountered upon birth. As previously stated, manual resuscitators are the first-line device recommended for emergency artificial ventilation of critical care patients, and are thus used not only throughout hospitals but also in out-of-hospital care venues by firefighters, paramedics and outpatient clinic personnel.

Inability of Professional Providers to use Manual Resuscitators within Established Safety Guidelines

Manual resuscitators have no built-in tidal volume control – the amount of air used to force-inflate the lungs during each breath depends entirely on how much the operator squeezes the bag. In response to the dangers associated with use of manual resuscitators, specific guidelines from the American Heart Association and European Resuscitation Council were issued that specify recommended maximal tidal volumes (or breath sizes) and ventilation rates safe for patients. While no studies are known that have assessed the frequency of complications and/or deaths due to uncontrolled manual resuscitator use, numerous peer-reviewed studies have found that, despite established safety guidelines, the incidence of provider over-inflation with manual resuscitators continues to be "endemic" and unrelated to provider training or skill level. Another clinical study found "the tidal volume delivered by a manual resuscitator shows large variations", concluding that "the manual resuscitator is not a suitable device for accurate ventilation." A separate assessment of another high-skilled group with frequent emergency use of manual resuscitators (ambulance paramedics) found that "Despite seemingly adequate training, EMS personnel consistently hyperventilated patients during out-of-hospital CPR", with the same research group concluding that "Unrecognized and inadvertent hyperventilation may be contributing to the currently dismal survival rates from cardiac arrest." A peer-reviewed study published in 2012 assessed the possible incidence of uncontrolled over-inflation in newborn neonates, finding that "a large discrepancy between the delivered and the current guideline values was observed for all parameters," and that "regardless of profession or handling technique ... 88.4% delivered excessive pressures, whereas ... 73.8% exceeded the recommended range of volume", concluding that "the great majority of participants from all professional groups delivered excessive pressures and volumes." A further examination has recently been made to assess whether a solution to the over-ventilation problem may lie with use of pediatric-sized manual resuscitators in adults or use of more advanced flow-inflation (or "Mapleson C") versions of manual resuscitators: while "the paediatric self-inflating bag delivered the most guideline-consistent ventilation", it did not lead to full guideline compliance as "participants hyperventilated patients' lungs in simulated cardiac arrest with all three devices."

Guideline Non-compliance Due to Excessive Rate Versus Excessive Lung Inflation

"Hyperventilation" can be achieved through delivery of (1) too many breaths per minute; (2) breaths that are too large and exceed the patient's natural lung capacity; or (3) a combination of both. With use of manual resuscitators, neither rate nor inflating volumes can be physically controlled through built-in safety adjustments within the device itself, and as highlighted above, studies show providers frequently exceed designated safety guidelines for both ventilation rate (10 breaths per minute) and volume (5–7 mL / kg body weight) as outlined by the American Heart Association and European Resuscitation Council. Numerous studies have concluded that ventilation at rates in excess of current guidelines are capable of interfering with blood flow during cardiopulmonary resuscitation, however the pre-clinical experiments associated with these findings involved delivery of inspiratory volumes in excess of current guidelines (e.g., they assessed the effects of hyperventilation via both excessive rate and excessive volumes simultaneously). A more recent study published in 2012 expanded knowledge on this topic by evaluating the separate effects of (1) isolated excessive rate with guideline-compliant inspiratory volumes; (2) guideline-compliant rate with excessive inspiratory volumes; and (3) combined guideline non-compliance with both excessive rate and volume. This study found that excessive rate more than triple the current guideline (e.g., 33 breaths per minute) may not interfere with CPR when inspiratory volumes are delivered within guideline-compliant levels, suggesting that ability to keep breath sizes within guideline limits may individually mitigate clinical dangers of excessive rate. It was also found that when guideline-excessive tidal volumes were delivered, changes in blood flow were observed that were transient at low ventilation rates but sustained when both tidal volumes and rates were simultaneously excessive, suggesting that guideline-excessive tidal volume is the principal mechanism of side effects, with ventilation rate acting as a multiplier of these effects. Consistent with previous studies where both excessive rate and volumes were found to produce side effects of blood flow interference during CPR, a complicating factor may be inadequate time to permit full expiration of oversized breaths in between closely spaced high-rate breaths, leading to the lungs never being permitted to fully exhale between ventilations (also called "stacking" of breaths). A recent advancement in the safety of manual ventilation may be the growing use of time-assist devices that emit an audible and/or visual metronome tone or flashing light at the proper guideline-designated rate interval for breath frequency; one study found these devices may lead to near 100% guideline compliance for ventilation rate. While this advancement appears to provide a solution to the "rate problem" associated with guideline-excessive manual resuscitator use, it may not address the "volume problem" which may continue to make manual resuscitators a patient hazard (as complications can still occur from over-inflation even when rate is delivered within guidelines).

Currently the only devices that can deliver pre-set, physician-prescribed inflation volumes reliably within safety guidelines are mechanical ventilators that require an electrical power source and/or a source of compressed oxygen, a higher level of training to operate, and typically cost hundreds to thousands of dollars more than a disposable manual resuscitator.

Additional Components / Features

Filters

A filter is sometimes placed between the mask and the bag (before or after the valve) to prevent contamination of the bag.

Positive End-expiratory Pressure

Some devices have PEEP valve connectors, for better positive airway pressure maintenance.

Medication Delivery

A covered port may be incorporated into the valve assembly to allow inhalatory medicines to be injected into the airflow, which may be particularly effective in treating patients in respiratory arrest from severe asthma.

Airway Pressure Port

A separate covered port may be included into the valve assembly to enable a pressure-monitoring device to be attached, enabling rescuers to continuously monitor the amount of positive-pressure being generated during forced lung inflation.

Pressure Relief Valves

A pressure relief valve (often known as a "pop-up valve") is typically included in pediatric versions and some adult versions, the purpose of which is to prevent accidental over-pressurization of the lungs. A bypass clip is usually incorporated into this valve assembly in case medical needs call for inflation at a pressure beyond the normal cutoff of the pop-up valve.

Device Storage Features

Some bags are designed to collapse for storage. A bag not designed to store collapsed may lose elasticity when stored compressed for long periods, reducing its effectiveness. The collapsible design has longitudinal scoring so that the bag collapses on the scoring "pivot point," opposite to the direction of normal bag compression.

Manual Resuscitator Alternatives

In a hospital, long-term mechanical ventilation is provided by using a more complex, automated ventilator. However a frequent use of a manual resuscitator is to temporarily provide manual ventilation whenever troubleshooting of the mechanical ventilator is needed, if the ventilator circuit needs to be changed, or if there is a loss of electrical power or source of compressed air and/or oxygen.

A rudimentary type of mechanical ventilator device that has the advantage of not needing electricity is a flow-restricted, oxygen-powered ventilation device (FROPVD). These are similar to manual resuscitators in that oxygen is pushed through a mask to force-inflate the patient's lungs, but unlike a manual resuscitator where the pressure used to force-inflate the patient's lungs comes from a person manually squeezing a bag, with the FROPVD the pressure needed to force-inflate the lungs comes directly from a pressurized oxygen cylinder. These devices will stop functioning when the compressed oxygen tank becomes depleted.

Types of Manual Resuscitators

- Self-inflating bags: This type of manual resuscitator is the standard design most often used in both in-hospital and out-of-hospital settings. The material used for the bag-portion of a self-inflating manual resuscitator has a "memory", meaning after it is manually compressed it will automatically re-expand on its own in between breaths (drawing in air for the next breath). These devices can be used alone (thus delivering room-air) or can be used in connection with an oxygen source to deliver nearly 100% oxygen. As a result of these features, this type of manual resuscitator is appropriate for in-hospital use and in out-of-hospital settings (e.g., ambulances).

- Flow-inflating bags: Also termed "anesthesia bags," these are a specialized form of manual resuscitator with a bag-portion that is flaccid and does not re-inflate on its own. This necessitates an external flow source of pressurized inflation gas for the bag to inflate; once inflated the provider can manually squeeze the bag or, if the patient is breathing on his/her own, the patient can inhale directly through the bag itself. These types of manual resuscitators are used extensively during anesthesia induction and recovery, and are often attached to anesthesia consoles so anesthesia gases can be used to ventilate the patient. They are primarily utilized by anesthesiologists administering general anesthesia, but also during some in-hospital emergencies which may involve anesthesiologists or respiratory therapists. They are not typically used outside hospital settings.As per a recent Indian study, these flow inflation bags can also be used to provide CPAP in spontaneously breathing children.

Cervical Collar

A cervical collar, also known as a neck brace, is a medical device used to support a person's neck. It is also used by emergency personnel for those who have had traumatic head or neck injuries, and can be used to treat chronic medical conditions.

Whenever people have a traumatic head or neck injury, they may have a cervical fracture. This makes them at high risk for spinal cord injury, which could be exacerbated by movement of the person and could lead to paralysis or death. A common scenario for this injury would be a person suspected of having whiplash because of a car accident. In order to prevent further injury, such people may have a collar placed by medical professionals until X-rays can be taken to determine if a cervical spine fracture exists. The cervical collar only stabilizes the top seven vertebrae, C1 through C7. (Other immobilizing devices such as a Kendrick Extrication Device or a backboard can be used to stabilize the remainder of the spinal column.)

Cervical collars are also used therapeutically to help realign the spinal cord and relieve pain, although they are usually not worn for long periods of time. Another use of the cervical collar is for strains, sprains or whiplash. If pain is persistent, the collar might be required to remain attached to help in the healing process. A person may also need a cervical collar, or may require a halo fixation device to support the neck during recovery after surgery such as cervical spinal fusion.

Types

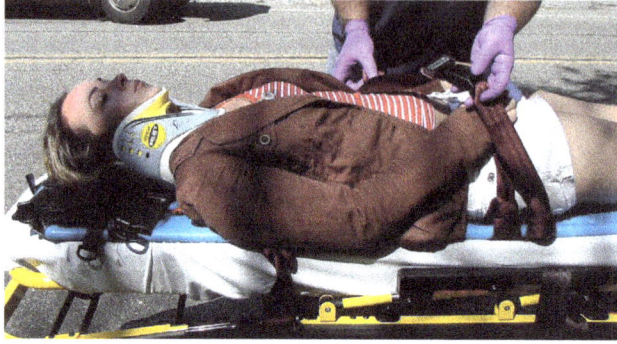

A neck collar being placed on a girl by emergency services.

A soft collar is fairly flexible and is the least limiting but can carry a high risk of further breakage, especially in people with osteoporosis. It can be used for minor injuries or after healing has allowed the neck to become more stable.

A range of manufactured rigid collars are also used, usually comprising (a) a firm plastic bi-valved shell secured with Velcro straps and (b) removable padded liners. The most frequently prescribed are the Aspen, Malibu, Miami J, and Philadelphia collars. All these can be used with additional chest and head extension pieces to increase stability.

Cervical collars are incorporated into rigid braces that constrain the head and chest together. Examples include the Sterno-Occipital Mandibular Immobilization Device (SOMI), Lerman Minerva and Yale types. Special cases, such as very young children or non-cooperative adults, are sometimes still immobilized in medical plaster of paris casts, such as the Minerva cast.

Sport

In high-risk motorsports such as Motocross, go-kart racing and speed-boat racing, racers often wear a protective collar to avoid whiplash and other neck injuries.

Designs range from simple foam collars to complex composite devices.

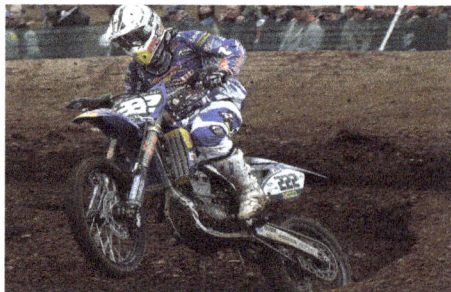

A motocross rider wearing a sports neck brace

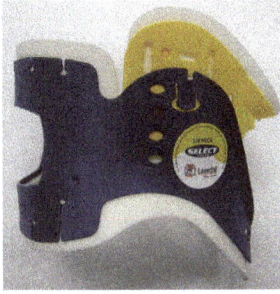
Side view of a cervical collar

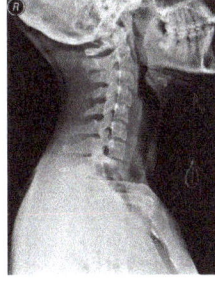
Side view X-ray of the neck with a cervical collar.

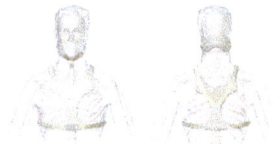
Sterno-Occipital Mandibular Immobilizer (SOMI)
SOMI brace.

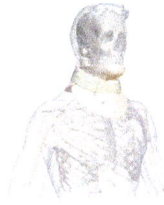
Cervical Collar
Cervical collar.

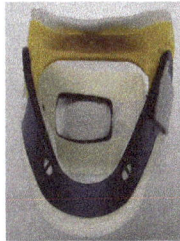
Front view of a cervical collar. The opening |provides anterior access to the neck for a cricothyrotomy or tracheotomy.

Nitrous Oxide (Medication)

Nitrous oxide, sold under the brand name Entonox among others, is an inhaled gas used as a pain medication and together with other medications for anesthesia. Common uses include during childbirth, following trauma, and as part of end of life care. Onset of effect is typically within half a minute and lasts for about a minute.

There are few side effects, other than vomiting, with short term use. With long term use anemia or numbness may occur. It should always be given with at least 21% oxygen. It is not recommended in people with a bowel obstruction or pneumothorax. Use in the early part of pregnancy is not recommended. Breastfeeding can occur following use.

Nitrous oxide was discovered between 1772 and 1793 and used for anesthesia in 1844. It is on the World Health Organization's List of Essential Medicines, the most effective and safe medicines needed in a health system. It often comes as a 50/50 mixture with oxygen. Devices with a demand valve are available for self-administration. The setup and maintenance is relatively expensive for developing countries.

Medical uses

Nitrous oxide (N_2O) is itself active (does not require any changes in the body to become active), and so has an onset in roughly the lung–brain circulation time. This gives it a peak action 30 seconds after the start of administration; Entonox should thus be used accordingly, i.e. inhalation should start 30 seconds before a contraction becomes painful in labour. It is removed from the body unchanged via the lungs, and does not accumulate under normal conditions, explaining the rapid offset of around 60 seconds.

Nitrous oxide is more soluble than oxygen and nitrogen, so will tend to diffuse into any air spaces within the body. This makes it dangerous to use in patients with pneumothorax or those who have recently been scuba diving, and there are cautions over its use with any bowel obstruction.

Its analgesic effect is strong (equivalent to 15 mg of subcutaneous route morphine) and characterised by rapid onset and offset, i.e. it is very fast-acting and wears off very quickly.

Contraindications

N_2O should not be used in patients with bowel obstruction, pneumothorax, middle ear or sinus disease, and should also not be used on any patient who has been scuba diving within the preceding 24 hours or in violently disturbed psychiatric patients. There are also clinical cautions in place for the first two trimesters of pregnancy and in patients with decreased levels of consciousness.

Composition

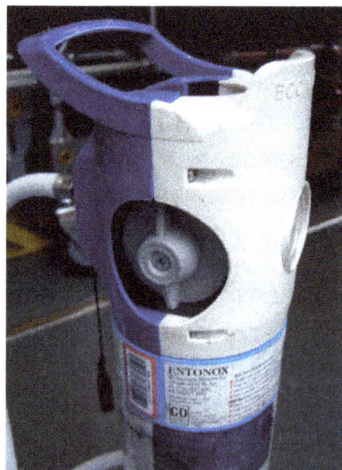

Distinct blue and white cap of an Entonox cylinder

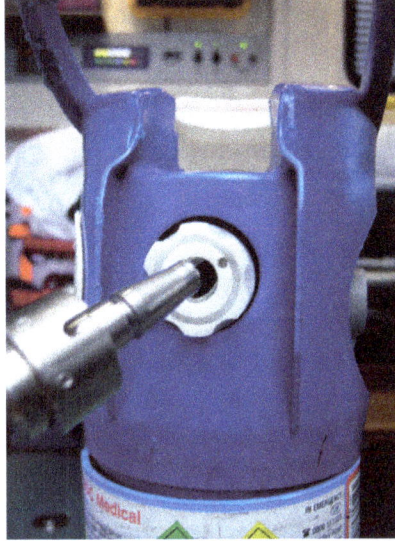

Typical Schrader valve attachment, making the gas usable only with demand based giving sets

The gas is a mixture of half nitrous oxide (N_2O or laughing gas) and half oxygen (O_2). The ability to combine N_2O (nitrous oxide is the common name; dinitrogen monoxide, systematic name) and oxygen at high pressure while remaining in the gaseous form is caused by the Poynting effect (after John Henry Poynting, an English physicist).

The Poynting effect involves the dissolution of gaseous O_2 when bubbled through liquid N_2O, with vaporisation of the liquid to form a gaseous O_2/N_2O mixture.

Inhalation of pure N_2O over a continued period would deprive the patient of oxygen, but the 50% oxygen content prevents this from occurring. The two gases will separate at low temperatures (<4 °C), which would permit administration of hypoxic mixtures. Therefore, it is not given from a cold cylinder without being shaken (usually by cylinder inversion) to remix the gases.

Administration

The gas is self-administered through a demand valve, using a mouthpiece, bite block or face mask. Self-administration of Entonox is safe because if enough is inhaled to start to induce anaesthesia, the patient becomes unable to hold the valve, and so will drop it and soon exhale the residual gas. This means that unlike other anaesthetic gases, it does not require the presence of an anaesthetist for administration. The 50% oxygen in Entonox ensures the patient will have sufficient oxygen in their system for a short period of apnea (or apnoea) to be safe.

History

Pure N_2O was first used as a medical analgesic in December 1844, when Horace Wells made the first 12–15 dental operations with the gas in Hartford..

Its debut as a generally accepted method, however, came in 1863, when Gardner Quincy Colton introduced it more broadly at all the Colton Dental Association clinics, that he founded in New Haven and New York City.

The first devices used in dentistry to administer the gas consisted of a simple breathing bag made of rubber cloth.

Breathing the pure gas often caused hypoxia (oxygen insufficiency) and sometimes death by asphyxiation. Eventually practitioners became aware of the need to provide at least 21% oxygen content in the gas (the same percentage as in air). In 1911, the anaesthetist Arthur Ernest Guedel first described the use of self-administration of a nitrous oxide and oxygen mix. It was not until 1961 that the first paper was published by Michael Tunstall and others, describing the administration of a pre-mixed 50:50 nitrous oxide and oxygen mix, which led to the commercialisation of the product.

Today the nitrous oxide is administered in hospitals by a relative analgesia machine, which includes several improvements such as flowmeters and constant-flow regulators, an anaesthetic vaporiser, a medical ventilator, and a scavenger system, and delivers a precisely dosed and breath-actuated flow of nitrous oxide mixed with oxygen.

The machine used in dentistry is much simpler, and is meant to be used by the patient in a fully conscious state. The gas is delivered through a demand-valve inhaler over the nose, which will only release gas when the patient inhales through it.

Society and Culture

Nitronox is a registered trademark of BOC. It is also colloquially known as "gas and air".

Research

Investigational trials show potential for antidepressant applications of N_2O, especially for treatment-resistant forms of depression, and it is rapid-acting.

Non-pneumatic Anti-shock Garment

The non-pneumatic anti-shock garment (NASG) is a low-technology first-aid device used to treat hypovolemic shock. Its efficacy for reducing maternal deaths due to obstetrical hemorrhage is being researched. Obstetrical hemorrhage is heavy bleeding of a woman during or shortly after a pregnancy. Current estimates suggest over 300,000 women die every year, of which 99% occurs in developing countries, most of which are preventable. Many women in resource-poor settings deliver far from health-care facilities. Once hemorrhage has been identified, many women die before reaching or receiving adequate treatment. The NASG can be used to keep women alive until they can get the treatment they need.

Background

Every year, an estimated 342,900 women die from complications of pregnancy and childbirth, 99% of these deaths occur in developing countries. Worldwide, for every 100,000 live births, about 251 women die. In some industrialized countries such as the U.S, this is 13 deaths for every 100,000 live babies born with American women having a lifetime risk of 1 in 2,100 of dying from childbirth related complications. However, in some countries, such as Afghanistan up to 1,600 women die for every 100,000 live births and women have a 1 in 11 lifetime risk of maternal death.

For every woman who dies, there are 30 women who suffer a disability as a result of pregnancy or childbirth related complications (a maternal morbidity) and 10 who experience a 'near miss mortality' (a life-threatening obstetric complication). Morbidities can be serious, lifelong ailments which compromise a woman's health, productivity, quality of life, family health and ability to participate in community life. If a mother dies after childbirth, the newborn is ten times more likely to die before the age of two, other children are more likely to suffer from decreased nutrition and decreased schooling. Many motherless families find it difficult to survive, often with older children having to drop out of school in order to work to help support the family or being sent to live with a relatives intact family. In addition to this, maternal and newborn deaths are estimated to cost the world $15 billion in lost productivity annually, with maternal health proven to support a country's economic growth and cut poverty. Maternal death and disability is a human rights issue. It also means hardships and loss of productivity for families, communities and nations. This is of such great concern that in 2000, world leaders decided that improving maternal health should be one of the 8 Millennium Development Goals for the international community.

The leading cause of maternal mortality (deaths from pregnancy and childbirth related complications) is obstetric hemorrhage in which a woman bleeds heavily, most often immediately after giving birth. A woman dies every 4 minutes from this kind of complication. A woman can bleed to death in two hours or less, and in rural areas, where hospitals may be days away, this leaves little hope for women suffering from hemorrhage. Also, in areas that have limited resources, clinics and hospitals might not have the staff or supplies needed to save a woman's life. Women die waiting for treatment.

There are some emerging technologies which are currently being researched and implemented that seek to prevent these unnecessary deaths. One of these is the NASG which is a low-technology first-aid device that can be placed around the lower body of a woman who has gone into shock from obstetric bleeding. This garment decreases blood loss, recovers women from shock and keeps them alive while they are traveling to a hospital or awaiting treatment.

History

In the 1900s an inflatable pressure suit was developed by George Crile. It was used to maintain blood pressure during surgery. In the 1940s and after undergoing numerous modifications, the suit was refined for use as an anti-gravity suit (G-suit). Further modification led to its use in the Vietnam War for resuscitating and stabilizing soldiers with traumatic injuries before and during transportation. In the 1970s the G-suit was modified into a half-suit which became known as MAST (Military anti-shock trousers) or PASG (Pneumatic Anti-Shock Garment). During the 1980s the PASG garment became used more and more by emergency rescue services to stabilize patients with shock due to lower body hemorrhage. During the 1990s the PASG was added to the American College of Obstetrics and Gynecology, making it part of the recommended treatment for use by obstetricians and gynecologists in the USA. However, it was removed from the guidelines later and is no longer on the ACOG guidelines.

From the 1970s, NASA/Ames was involved in developing a non-pneumatic version of the anti-shock garment. This was originally used for hemophiliac children, but has since been developed into the garment known as the Non-pneumatic Anti-Shock Garment (NASG).

The non-pneumatic anti-shock garment is now off-patent and produced in several different locations.

The use of the garment for obstetrical hemorrhage in low-resource settings began in 2002 when Dr. Carol Brees and Dr. Paul Hensleigh introduced the garment into a hospital in Pakistan and reported on a case series of its use.

Suellen Miller and colleagues in Mexico, Egypt and Nigeria have completed studies of the NASG (also named the LifeWrap) for obstetric hemorrhage in hospitals in these countries with studies ongoing at primary health care centers in Zambia and Zimbabwe. An implementation program with the NASG as part of a Continuum of Care for Post-Partum Hemorrhage (CCPPH) has been underway since 2008 in India, Nigeria, Tanzania and Peru. The NGO Pathfinder International is the lead implementing organization on the CCPPH project. Dr. Suellen Miller has done extensive clinical trials with the device as an obstetric first aid. The U.S. based non-profit organization, Pathfinder International has worked on developing the Continuum of Care model.

How it Works

The non-pneumatic anti-shock garment is a simple neoprene and Velcro device that looks like the bottom half of a wetsuit cut into segments. It can be used to treat shock, resuscitate, stabilize and prevent further bleeding in women with obstetric hemorrhage.

When in shock, the brain, heart and lungs are deprived of oxygen because blood accumulates in the lower abdomen and legs. The NASG reverses shock by returning blood to the heart, lungs and brain. This restores the woman's consciousness, pulse and blood pressure. Additionally, the NASG decreases bleeding from the parts of the body compressed under it.

Mechanisms of action are based upon laws of physics. Recent research has identified that the pressure applied by the NASG serves to significantly increase the resistive index of the internal iliac artery (which is responsible for supplying the majority of blood flow to the uterus via the uterine arteries). Another recent study has shown the NASG to decrease blood flow in the distal aorta.

After a simple training session, anyone can put the garment on a bleeding woman. Once her bleeding is controlled, she can be safely transported to a referral hospital for emergency obstetrical care.

The non-pneumatic anti-shock garment is light, flexible and comfortable for the wearer. It has been designed to allow perineal access so that examinations and vaginal procedures can be performed without it being removed. Upon application a patient's vital signs are often quickly restored and consciousness regained. It is extremely important not to remove the NASG before a woman receives IV fluids, blood and before all vital signs are restored. Early removal can be dangerous and even fatal.

Research and Implementation

In Egypt and Nigeria, in separate and combined analyses, findings showed that women treated with the NASG fared much better than women who were not treated with the NASG. Results showed significant reductions in blood loss, rate of emergency hysterectomy and incidence of morbidity and mortality. Analyses examining the use of the NASG on cases of uterine atony, postpartum hemorrhage, and non-atonic etiologies (ante and postpartum) found similar results. Other analyses found that the NASG additionally resulted in a more rapid recovery from shock, helped women overcome treatment delays and had a similarly strong ameliorative effect on women in severe shock.

A combined analysis on 1442 women recently published, examined the effect of the NASG on women with obstetric hemorrhage. Despite being in a worse condition at study entry, negative outcomes were significantly reduced in the NASG phase: mean measured blood loss decreased from 444 mL to 240 mL ($p<0.001$), maternal mortality decreased from 6.3% to 3.5% (RR 0.56, 95% CI 0.35–0.89), severe morbidities from 3.7% to 0.7% (RR 0.20, 95% CI 0.08–0.50), and emergency hysterectomy from 8.9% to 4.0% (RR 0.44, 0.23–0.86). In multiple logistic regression, there was a 55% reduced odds of mortality during the NASG phase (aOR 0.45, 0.27–0.77). The number needed to treat (NNT) to prevent either mortality or severe morbidity was 18 (12–36).

Qualitative research in Mexico and Nigeria has examined acceptance of the NASG and found that overall, there were positive reactions to the garment as a relevant technology for saving women's lives.

Research is currently ongoing in Zambia and Zimbabwe to investigate whether the NASG is more successful if implemented at primary health care facilities where hemorrhage is first identified.

In 2012, the World Health Organization included the NASG in its recommendations for the treatment of postpartum hemorrhage.

Splint (Medicine)

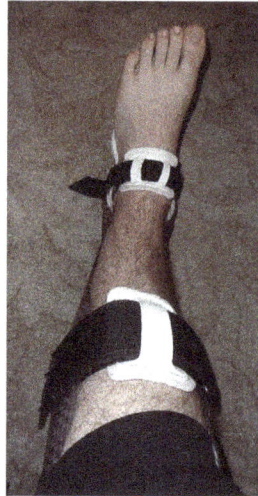

An Ankle Foot Orthosis (AFO) is a type of splint used to support the foot and ankle.

A splint is a device used for support or immobilization of a limb or the spine. It can be used in multiple situations, including temporary immobilization of potentially broken bones or damaged joints and support for joints during activity.

Uses

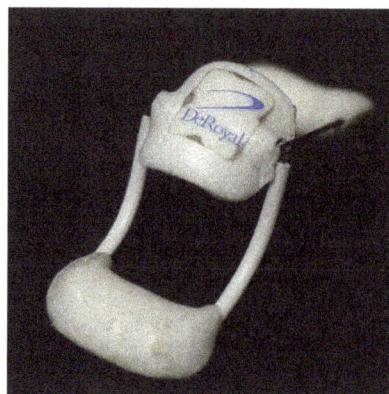

Capener finger splint

- By the emergency medical services or by volunteer first responders, to temporarily immobilize a fractured limb before transportation;

- By allied health professionals such as occupational therapists, physiotherapists and orthotists, to immobilize an articulation (e.g. the knee) that can be freed while not standing (e.g. during sleep);

- By athletic trainers to immobilize an injured bone or joint to facilitate safer transportation of the injured person; or

- By emergency room (ER) physicians to stabilize fractures or sprains until follow-up appointment with an orthopedist.

Commonly Used Splints

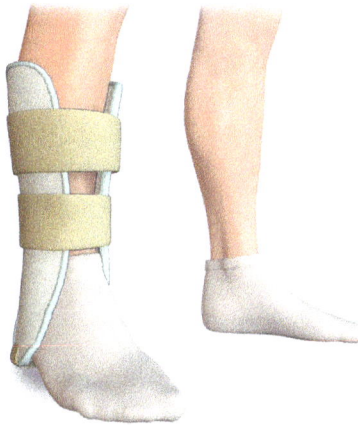

Ankle Stirrup Splint

Illustration of an Ankle Stirrup Splint

- Ankle Stirrup - Used for the ankles

- Finger Splints - Used for the fingers

- Nasal splint

- Posterior Lower Leg

- Posterior Full Leg

- Posterior Elbow

- Sugar Tong - Used for the forearm or wrist. They are named "sugar-tong" due to their long, U-shaped characteristics, similar to a type of utensil used to pick up sugar cubes

- Thumb Spica - Used for the thumb

- Ulnar Gutter - Used for the forearm to the palm

- Volar Wrist Splint - Used for the wrist

- Wrist/arm splint - Used for the wrist or arm

Assisted Cough Technique

Commonly used after surgery to provide support to an incised area and decrease pain on coughing.

While the patient attempts to cough the area is braced by the patient (or assistant) using pillow, folded blanket or extended hand placed over the incision.

Gentle pressure is applied for bracing only during the attempt to cough.

Different forms of the splint have been used sparingly throughout history; however, the splint gained great popularity as a medical device during the French and Indian War. Generally consisting of two small wooden planks, the splint was commonly tied around the fracture with rope, cloth, or even rawhide during frontier times in American history. To this day, the splint is commonly used to secure small fractures and breaks.

Vacuum Mattress

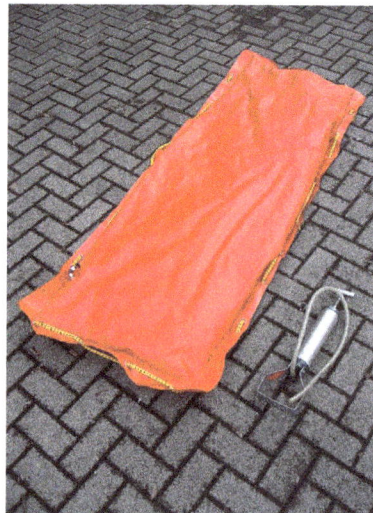

Vacuum mattress and its manual pump

A vacuum mattress, or vacmat, is a medical device used for the immobilisation of patients, especially in case of a vertebra, pelvis or limb trauma (especially for femur trauma). It is also used for manual transportation of patients for short distances (it replaces the stretcher). It was invented by Loed and Haederlé, who called it "shell" mattress (*matelas coquille* in French).

Operation

A vacuum mattress consists of a sealed air-tight (typically polymer) bag enclosing small beads (typically polystyrene balls) and fitted with one or more valves. While at ambient air pressure, the beads free to move, but when the mattress has been moulded and the air evacuated, external atmospheric pressure locks the beads in place (jamming) and the mattress becomes rigid.

When used medically this principle allows a patient is put on the mattress (e.g. with a scoop stretcher), the sides of the mattress arranged around the patient and when the air inside is evacuated the mattress forms a conformal cradle allowing an injury to be stabilised, straps fastened, and the patient protected sufficiently well that they can be transported.

For this reason the bag is typically bigger than an adult human body (though the same principle may be employed to create an 'instant' cast to stabilise an injured limb. In use a sheet is usually put on the vacuum mattress to:

- Protect the mattress from penetration, preserving the integrity of the air-tight bag. (The casualty may have broken glass on their clothes or be wearing jewellery that might puncture the mattress.)

- Avoid direct contact of the skin with plastic (The patient may be releasing body fluids.)

- To assist in transferring the patient at the emergency room.

Medical Uses

The full spine immobilisation (splint) is performed with:

- a rigid cervical collar

- a vacuum mattress

- a stretcher under it (the longitudinal stiffness of the mattress alone is not sufficient).

Preparation of the Vacuum Mattress

The vacuum mattress is put on a stretcher or possibly on a long spine board. The straps are put under the mattress, along its side, so they do not reach the ground. Then, the polystyrene balls are distributed evenly through the mattress by shaking its surface. (A section with fewer balls would be less rigid, conversely if balls are concentrated at any given point this becomes more rigid.) A sheet is put on the mattress, folded so it will be possible to pull it to wrap the casualty into using an S-fold and finally a team member should double-check the pump (manual or electrical) is set to either pump air out of the bag.

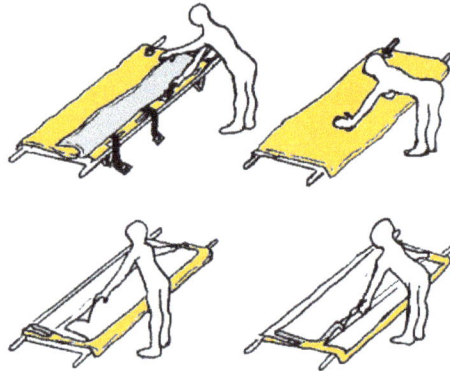

Preparation of the vacuum mattress

Moulding the Mattress

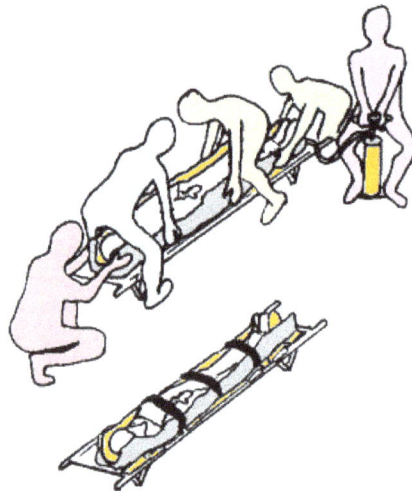

Moulding of the vacuum mattress

There are three ways to put the casualty on the vacuum mattress:

- lifting the casualty and pushing the stretcher under it. This method requires a minimum of five team members (four lifting and one pushing the stretcher) and should be used when a spine or a pelvis trauma are suspected;

- the casualty is lifted with a scoop stretcher. The scoop stretcher is put on the mattress and opened to release the casualty;

- the casualty is lifted on a long spine board. The board is put on the mattress and the casualty is lifted (best with four team members) and one team member removes the board.

In all cases, the vacuum valve is up and at the feet of the casualty.

Once the casualty is on the mattress, the sheet is wrapped around him/her and the sides of the mattress are folded against their body. The top of the head must be kept clear (the mattress could retract when pumping out the air and thus compress the spine). The air is pumped until the mattress is rigid, then the valve is closed and the straps are fastened.

When only three team members are available and there is no scoop stretcher, the following procedure can be used:

1. the vacuum mattress is put besides the casualty, on a protecting ground sheet, and partially depressed (three manual pumping) to make it more rigid and thinner. A sheet is put on the mattress, closer to the casualty;

2. the casualty is put on their side, with a procedure that is similar to the recovery position;

3. the team member at the legs pushes the mattress against the back of the casualty. The ground sheet helps to slide the mattress on the floor;

4. the casualty is put on their back, overlapping the side of the mattress;

5. the casualty is centred on the mattress; the sheet helps sliding the casualty on the mattress;

6. the straps are tied to mould the mattress. The team leader moulds the sides of the head manually;

7. the air is pumped;

8. a long spine board is placed along the axis of the mattress. Two team members face each other and hold the mattress's handles at the head and at the thighs. They lift a few centimetres, the ground sheet is removed and the board is slid under the mattress to ensure longitudinal rigidity;

9. the board can then be lifted (with the mattress on it), and put on the stretcher.

While the lifting methods can induce a flexing of the spine, this rolling method can be hazardous for several reasons: the risk of a torsion of the spine when rolling, the risk when sliding the casualty on the mattress, the risk of anteversion of the hips (and thus of flexing of the spine) due to the weight of the legs when lifting the mattress to slide the board.

Advantages and Disadvantages

The vacuum mattress is an alternative to the use of a long spine board. Its advantages are:

- Comfort.

- Being adaptable to all traumas (included spinal and femoral traumas).

- The patient is held more securely.

- The patient is more easily transported short distances provided sufficient team members (typically six) are available, and in confined spaces compared to a conventional stretcher.

Its drawbacks include:

- Relatively fragile (useless unless a perfect vacuum is maintained).

- Increased cost relative to a traditional long spine board

- The time taken to evacuate the bag compared to readily-available standard spinal board.

References

- Sen, Ayan (2005). "Spinal Immobilisation in Prehospital Trauma Patient". Journal of Emergency Primary Health Care. 3 (3). ISSN 1447-4999

- The trauma handbook of the Massachusetts General Hospital. Philadelphia: Lippincott Williams & Wilkins. 2004. p. 37. ISBN 9780781745963

- Hart, AP; Azar, VJ; Hart, KR; Stephens, BG (2005). "Autopsy artifact created by the Revivant AutoPulse resuscitation device". Journal of forensic sciences. 50 (1): 164–8. doi:10.1520/jfs2004155. PMID 15831013

- "Cardiopulmonary Resuscitation (CPR) Statistics". American Red Cross. Archived from the original on 19 November 2008. Retrieved 2008-10-27

- ."The use of the spinal board after the pre-hospital phase of trauma management". Emergency Medical Journal. 18 (1): 51–54. 2001. doi:10.1136/emj.18.1.51

- Mistovich, Joseph J.; Brent Q. Hafen; Keith J Karren (2000). Brady Prehospital Emergency Care (6 ed.). Upper Saddle River, NJ: Prentice-Hall. p. 662. ISBN 0-8359-6064-1

- Silbergleit R, Lee DC, Blank-Ried C, McNamara RM. Sudden severe barotrauma from self-inflating bag devices. Journal of Trauma 1996: 40:320–322

- "Miracle man comes back 'from the dead' after 3.5 hours - medical skill and high tec machine save him". Daily Mirror. 2011-01-14. Archived from the original on 2012-02-13. Retrieved 2013-02-07

- Morrissey, J (Mar 2013). "Spinal immobilization. Time for a change.". JEMS : a journal of emergency medical services. 38 (3): 28–30, 32–6, 38–9. PMID 23717917

- Mistovich, Joseph J.; Brent Q. Hafen; Keith J Karren (2000). Brady Prehospital Emergency Care (6 ed.). Upper Saddle River, NJ: Prentice-Hall. p. 662. ISBN 0-8359-6064-1

- "WHO recommendations for the prevention and treatment of postpartum haemorrhage (2012)" (PDF). Retrieved 21 September 2013

- Lee HM, Cho KH, Choi YH, Yoon SY, Choi YH. Can you deliver accurate tidal volume by manual resuscitator. Emergency Medicine Journal 2008: 10:632–634

Permissions

All chapters in this book are published with permission under the Creative Commons Attribution Share Alike License or equivalent. Every chapter published in this book has been scrutinized by our experts. Their significance has been extensively debated. The topics covered herein carry significant information for a comprehensive understanding. They may even be implemented as practical applications or may be referred to as a beginning point for further studies.

We would like to thank the editorial team for lending their expertise to make the book truly unique. They have played a crucial role in the development of this book. Without their invaluable contributions this book wouldn't have been possible. They have made vital efforts to compile up to date information on the varied aspects of this subject to make this book a valuable addition to the collection of many professionals and students.

This book was conceptualized with the vision of imparting up-to-date and integrated information in this field. To ensure the same, a matchless editorial board was set up. Every individual on the board went through rigorous rounds of assessment to prove their worth. After which they invested a large part of their time researching and compiling the most relevant data for our readers.

The editorial board has been involved in producing this book since its inception. They have spent rigorous hours researching and exploring the diverse topics which have resulted in the successful publishing of this book. They have passed on their knowledge of decades through this book. To expedite this challenging task, the publisher supported the team at every step. A small team of assistant editors was also appointed to further simplify the editing procedure and attain best results for the readers.

Apart from the editorial board, the designing team has also invested a significant amount of their time in understanding the subject and creating the most relevant covers. They scrutinized every image to scout for the most suitable representation of the subject and create an appropriate cover for the book.

The publishing team has been an ardent support to the editorial, designing and production team. Their endless efforts to recruit the best for this project, has resulted in the accomplishment of this book. They are a veteran in the field of academics and their pool of knowledge is as vast as their experience in printing. Their expertise and guidance has proved useful at every step. Their uncompromising quality standards have made this book an exceptional effort. Their encouragement from time to time has been an inspiration for everyone.

The publisher and the editorial board hope that this book will prove to be a valuable piece of knowledge for students, practitioners and scholars across the globe.

Index